Gerald P. Mallon, DSW
Editor

Foundations
of Social Work Practice
with Lesbian and Gay Persons

Pre-publication
REVIEWS,
COMMENTARIES,
EVALUATIONS . . .

"**I** n a field exploding with new knowledge and ideas, Gerald Mallon's edited volume captures, synthesizes, deepens, and renders relevant for practice an extremely rich and complex body of theory and practice wisdom and, in the process, makes some original contributions of its own. Unified by systems and ecological metaphors, the chapters are uniformly excellent, up-to-date, and innovative, providing practitioners, educators, and students with an invaluable resource.

Knowledge for practice across system levels—with individuals, couples, families, groups, organizations, and communities—is addressed thoroughly and intelligently in highly accessible ways. Peg Hess and Howard Hess's chapter on the application of values and ethics in practice with lesbians and gays and Karina Walter's exploration of conflicting allegiances among lesbians and gays of color are particularly unique and compelling. I heartily suggest that this book become required reading for all social workers and other mental health practitioners."

Joan Laird, MS
Professor,
Smith College School
for Social Work,
Northhampton, MA

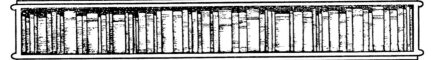

The Haworth Press, Inc.

Foundations
of Social Work Practice
with Lesbian and Gay Persons

THE HAWORTH PRESS
New, Recent, and Forthcoming Titles
of Related Interest

Foundations
of Social Work Practice
with Lesbian and Gay Persons

Gerald P. Mallon, DSW
Editor

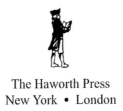

The Haworth Press
New York • London

The Haworth Press, Inc., 10 Alice Street, Binghamton, NY 13904-1580

Cover design by Monica Seifert.

Library of Congress Cataloging-in-Publication Data

Foundations of social work practice with lesbian and gay persons / Gerald P. Mallon, editor.
    p.   cm.
    Includes bibliographical references and index.
    ISBN 0-7890-0348-1 (alk. paper)
    1. Social work with gays—United States. 2. Gay men—Services for—United States. 3. Lesbians—Services for—United States. I. Mallon, Gerald P.
HV1449.F68 1998
362.8—dc21

                                      97-13382
                                           CIP

For Michael Rendino

CONTENTS

Chapter 6: Group Work Practice with Gay Men and Lesbians

George S. Getzel

Chapter 7: Social Work Practice with Gay Men and Lesbians Within Families

Gerald P. Mallon

ABOUT THE EDITOR

Gerald P. Mallon, DSW, is Assistant Professor in the School of Social Work at Columbia University. His research interests focus on the experiences of gay and lesbian children, youth, and families within the context of child welfare service delivery. Dr. Mallon is the author of the book *We Don't Exactly Get the Welcome Wagon: The Experiences of Gay and Lesbian Adolescents in Child Welfare Systems* (Columbia University Press).

Contributors

George A. Appleby, DSW, is Professor of Social Work at Southern Connecticut State University and a doctoral dissertation adviser for both Smith College and Union College.

Chrystal C. Ramirez Barranti, MSW, PhD, is Director of Continuing education and outreach, University of Georgia School of Social Work.

George S. Getzel, DSW, is Professor at the Hunter College School of Social Work.

Howard J. Hess, DSW, is Associate Dean and Professor at Fordham University School of Social Services.

Peg McCartt Hess, PhD, is Associate Dean and Associate Professor at Columbia University School of Social Work.

Joyce Hunter, DSW, is Director, Community Programs, at the HIV Center for Clinical and Behavioral Studies/New York State Psychiatric Institute.

Gerald P. Mallon, DSW, is Assistant Professor at Columbia University School of Social Work.

L. Donald McVinney, MSSW, CSW, CAC, is Director of Triangle Treatment, a gay, lesbian, bisexual, and transgender addictions treatment program at the Robinson Institute in New York, and Adjunct Professor at Columbia University School of Social Work.

Michael Shernoff, MSW, is in private practice in Manhattan, and is an adjunct lecturer at Hunter College Graduate School of Social Work.

Audrey I. Steinhorn, MSW, CSW, is in private practice in Manhattan and Poughkeepsie, New York.

Carol T. Tully, PhD, is Associate Professor at Tulane University School of Social Work.

Karina L. Walters, PhD, is Assistant Professor at Columbia University School of Social Work.

Foreword

In the 1970s, local bookstores boasted few if any books that dealt with the gay or lesbian experience. By the 1980s, what books there were that dealt with this population were found generally in small, local, homocentric book emporiums or in the back corner of the mall bookstore under a category called "Alternative Lifestyles." In the 1990s, not only has the number of books dealing with homosexuals and our lifestyles expanded greatly, but mainstream bookstores also jauntily include this content under the category of "Gay and Lesbian Studies." The development of social work content related to lesbians and gays has followed such a course as well. Moving from a few studies related to etiology in the 1950s; to more quantifiable research on psychological functioning in the 1960s; to quantifiable descriptive work dealing with social functioning in the 1970s; to studies and some books on life span development in the 1980s and 1990s; to more research and text related to clinical intervention, social workers continue to make great strides in the field of lesbian and gay studies. And social work books in this content area now have a presence among the bookshelves of mainstream bookstores as well.

Gerald Mallon and his colleagues continue this development of knowledge about social work practice with gay and lesbian persons in this volume. While gay and lesbian studies still must find general acceptance within the social work academic setting, the authors who are included in this book are willing to join those of us who have published in this field in the continuing struggle for equality. To become part of a movement that has yet to gain acceptance is indeed a brave thing; and yet, this willingness to challenge the system and advocate on behalf of those disenfranchised is at the core of social work's basic values and beliefs.

The focus of this book is on the pragmatic aspects of social work with gay and lesbian persons. The editor and his ten contributors present information related to how to deal with individuals who happen to be homocentric, as well as how to deal with lesbians and gays in the contexts of couples, families, groups, communities, and organizational structures. In doing so, the authors expand the social work knowledge base in a format that is instructive. Information related to the newly developing cyberspace makes this a timely contribution and one that is, at some levels, truly interactive.

One theme of the volume is the impact of institutional, individualized, and internal homophobia on social workers, their clients, and the institutions in which social workers practice. Homophobia can impair how social work professionals, their clients, and their agencies view each segment of the social environment and can prevent lesbian and gay clients from receiving adequate services. Through sensible strategies and case vignettes, the contributors to this edition provide much-needed information to help the social work practitioner deal with homophobia and heterocentrism.

In the emerging field of gay and lesbian social work studies, this work is one of the first of its kind to emerge in the 1990s. The eleven chapters presented include material related to micro, mezzo, and macro levels of social work; and the content related to the heterogeneity of the gay and lesbian population helps to make this a unique addition to the social work literature. Hopefully, this work will inspire others to join in the continuing development of content related to social work and lesbian and gay studies.

Carol T. Tully, PhD
Tulane University
New Orleans

Acknowledgments

Although the task of writing can be and often is a lonely endeavor, no one truly writes alone. One of the nicest things about completing a manuscript is having the opportunity to thank those who made the process more satisfying.

The idea for writing this book came from Ray Berger, who was one of the first social workers to write about social work practice with gay men and lesbians. His courage in writing about gay and lesbian persons, even though he was warned by friends and colleagues to "be careful," has allowed me and many others to write books that speak to the needs of persons whose voices have been silenced by the majority.

My immediate thanks are due next to those scholars and practitioners who agreed to author the works collected in this volume. One criterion for asking each of these professionals to participate in this project was that they be trained social work practitioners and educators. There have been several fine books that embraced a helping professional's perspective on gay and lesbian persons, but most were written by people who were not social workers. In writing this text about social work practice with gay and lesbian persons, it was important to me that all of the authors not only claim to have an understanding of a social work perspective, but that they actually practice from a social worker's perspective.

Michael Shernoff, one of the contributors to this volume, deserves special thanks from me not only because he has been a great friend, but because he is also a wonderful colleague who helped me during every step of this process. Michael is one of the most energetic people I have ever known. I have been genuinely inspired by his energy and commitment to challenging the social work profession, as he persistently urges our colleagues to provide competent practice with gay men and lesbians.

My colleagues at the Columbia University School of Social Work in New York, several of whom are contributors to this volume, have assisted me in completing this work by inviting me to a setting where the intellectual intensity and scholarly productivity are astounding. A recent text by the late Carol Meyer, a major anchor of social work education, and my other distinguished colleague Mark Mattaini, was the inspiration for writing this text. I learned a great deal from reading their book, *The Foundations of Social Work Practice,* and it provided a cogent and intelligent framework for writing this one. Two other colleagues merit acknowledgment: Peg Hess and Barbara Simon. Peg Hess, co-author of a chapter in this collection, has always been a wonderful role model for me and someone for whom I have the greatest admiration and respect. Professor Barbara Simon, my esteemed colleague at Columbia, is the most generous and unselfish associate with whom I have ever had the pleasure of working. She has not only been a great friend to me in this process, but has provided me with the level of intellectual stimulation and challenge that one would expect to find in the academy. I am proud to be a part of the Columbia University School of Social Work community.

Above all, I treasure the loving encouragement of my partner, Mike Rendino, who has provided me with a nutritive environment that has been conducive to my own growth as a person, and to my writing. His patience when I took "just an hour" to clean up a reference list or a few hours to fix a chapter was commendable. The kind of writing that academics need to do requires that we spend many hours away from our families. All the time I was writing, Mike was caring for our family: walking the dogs, cooking our meals, taking care of the kids, and much, much more. My thanks to Mike and to my family is inestimable.

Gerald P. Mallon, DSW

Chapter 1

Knowledge for Practice with Gay and Lesbian Persons

Gerald P. Mallon

"You are the first gay person whom I have ever met that appears to be happy about who you are," said a graduate social work student to me several years ago. She meant it as a compliment, but it made me sad that she thought all gay people were unhappy. "How many gay people do you know?" I asked in response to her comment. "Oh, you're the first," said she. I felt even worse. Even though this student had been exposed to one openly gay man, who happened to be her research professor, I could not help but ask myself how well she was being prepared to practice with gay men and lesbians in her field placement and in her course work. The answer, I knew, was that she was not being prepared at all. She had no courses that expanded her knowledge about the needs of gay men and lesbians; she had few, if any, readings assigned that addressed this content; and apart from her one experience with her openly gay professor, she had no practical experience in her professional training. It seemed woefully insufficient and somehow unethical to permit a student to graduate without any knowledge about the needs of this population. How were students, who would undoubtedly encounter gay men and lesbians in their professional lives, suppose to know how to practice with them? Unquestionably there was a need to address these issues with graduate students preparing for practice in a diverse world. Apart from its significance as a practice dilemma, this experience also illustrates an important truth about gay men and lesbians in contemporary society: that most people have little or no accurate knowledge about the lives of gay men and lesbians.

1

AN ECOLOGICAL APPROACH

The person:environment* perspective (Germain, 1991), utilized throughout this text as a framework for practice, has been a central influence on the profession's theoretical base and has usefulness and relevance as an approach to social work practice with gay men and lesbians. Germain and Gitterman (1996) underscore the point that disempowerment, which threatens the health, social well-being, and life of those who are oppressed, imposes enormous adaptive tasks on gay men and lesbians. An understanding of the destructive relationships that exist between gay men and lesbians and a predominantly heterocentric environment is integral to the process of developing practice knowledge about working with gay men and lesbians as clients. The purpose of this chapter, then, is to define and describe the knowledge base of practice with gay and lesbian persons and to review social work's response to the needs of this population.

What the social worker is supposed to do should dictate the boundaries of the profession's knowledge base, noted Meyer (1982). If social workers are supposed to be able to work with gay men and lesbians, then a knowledge base for practice with them must be within those boundaries. An organized knowledge base is crucial to any profession. Anyone, notes Mattaini (1995, p. 6) "can act." The professional, however, is expected to act deliberately, taking the steps that are likely to be most helpful, least intrusive, and most consistent with the person's welfare. Making a conscious determination about those choices requires an extensive knowledge base.

SOURCES OF KNOWLEDGE

In his chapter that focuses on the acquisition of knowledge for foundation practice, Mattaini (1995) identifies several key sources

---

*The conventional use of "person:environment" in the social work field represents the connection between the individual and his or her environmental context. Carel Germain, a pillar of social work education, felt so strongly about the interconnectedness of these concepts that she conceptualized them as inseparable, using a colon rather than a hyphen. I have chosen to use her concept in this text.

of knowledge that, in a modified version herein, provide a framework for this chapter's discussion on knowledge for practice with gay men and lesbians. Sources identified by Mattaini include (1) practice wisdom derived from narrative experiences of the profession and professional colleagues, (2) the personal experiences of the practitioner, (3) a knowledge of the professional literature, (4) a knowledge of history and current events, (5) research issues that inform practice (both qualitative and quantitative), (6) theoretical and conceptual analyses, and (7) information that is provided by the case itself. All of these, understood within an ecological framework of person:environment, with a consciousness of the reality of oppression in the lives of gay men and lesbians, is called upon to inform social work practice with gay and lesbian persons, and each source contributes to the development of the knowledge base of practice with this population.

PRACTICE WISDOM

Practice wisdom can be viewed as that which is derived from the narrative experiences of the profession, from both professional colleagues and from clients. Interest in narrative theory has grown in recent years, and the use of life stories in practice has in some organizations replaced elaborate, formalized intake histories. Life stories, which tend to be rich in detail, are usually obtained early in the work with a client and can be a useful means toward not only gathering important data to enhance one's knowledge base, but useful also in establishing a rapport and a trusting relationship with a gay or lesbian client. As the client tells and the worker listens empathically—that is, in the telling and the listening—the story gains personal and cultural meanings. This process, particularly with gay men and lesbians who have been oppressed, can be a healing process. It is, as Germain and Gitterman (1996, p. 145) put it, "our human way of finding meaning in life events, of explaining our life experience to ourselves and others, so that we can move on."

Over the years, several notable social work practitioners (English, 1996; MacPike, 1989; Muzio, 1996; Shernoff, 1991, 1996a) have provided excellent examples of the use of personal narrative as a means to enhance local knowledge that can guide practice (Hartman, 1992). Markowitz's (1991a) beautifully written and touching story of a lesbian daughter and her father as they struggle to forge a new understanding of one another is one almost perfect example of the power that personal narrative has to inform practice.

In addition to listening to the life stories of clients and the practice experiences of practitioners, social workers practicing with gay and lesbian persons can rely on rules that have been handed down by experienced practitioners. Heuristic practice, which can be described as principles to guide patterns of professional behavior and which has shaped and refined practice, may also serve as a model for other workers. The acquisition of group-specific language to guide practice, and a knowledge of the myths and stereotypes about gay men and lesbians can be extremely useful forms of heuristic practice. A glossary of terms and several of the most common myths about gay men and lesbians can be found in the appendix in this text. These fragments of practice wisdom can be valuable as a guide for practitioners interested in enhancing their practice knowledge base in working with gay men and lesbians.

PERSONAL EXPERIENCE

The personal experiences of practitioners is the second powerful force that guides knowledge development. Social workers are guided not only by their own personal experiences but also by a professional code of ethics (see McCartt Hess and Hess's chapter on values and ethics in this text). Most social workers base some of their knowledge about clients on integrated and synthesized events gathered from their own life experiences. Within the guidelines provided by the professions' code of ethics, basic interpersonal and problem-solving skills that social workers have developed throughout their lives are important means toward informing their practices.

It is a myth that most people do not know anyone who is gay or lesbian. Unquestionably, social workers who have a close friend or a family member who is openly gay or lesbian may have additional personal experiences that can assist them in guiding their practice with this population. Additionally, social workers who are themselves gay or lesbian will unquestionably have additional insights into gay and lesbian clients. However, being gay or lesbian alone does not provide a practitioner with a complete and full knowledge for practice with gay and lesbian clients. Individuals who are gay or lesbian may be at various stages of their own sexual identity development, and their knowledge may be, at best, incomplete.

Issues of self-disclosure become significant when a social worker has had personal experiences or shares something in common with a client, in this case a gay or lesbian identity. A gay or lesbian practitioner may find it helpful to disclose their orientation with a client who is struggling with whether or not to come out; but in other cases, the worker's disclosure could inhibit the client from sharing genuine feelings (Gartrell, 1994). Although self-disclosure can be useful in many cases (Cain, 1996; Rochlin, 1985), and while practitioners are using self-disclosure more than they did in the past, social workers need, at a minimum, close supervision and consultation to process these issues. Although personal experiences are key in knowledge development, social workers must always be in touch with their own feelings (Greene, 1994) and must remember that self-disclosure always has to do with the well-being of the client, not the practitioner.

HISTORY AND CURRENT EVENTS

Since practice is embedded in the broader social context of life, a knowledge of the social policies and shifting social forces is important for knowledge development and working with gay and lesbian persons. The media is an important source of information since historical events are most often documented in newspapers, in televised news reports, and in weekly and monthly magazines. Television talk shows and news journals are often less than objective and in many cases replete with inaccuracies; however, for many, these are the only sources of knowledge about gay men and lesbians and an important basis to work from, even in a professional context.

Recent media attention has thrust a variety of gay and lesbian issues out of the closet and into the homes of millions of people. Issues as varied as same-sex parental adoptions (Gay adoption,

1993, Judge lets, 1992); gay and lesbian partnership (Bennet, 1993; Schmalz, 1993c); gay and lesbian marriage (Zirin, 1996); benefits for same-sex partners (DePalma, 1992); gay and lesbian parents (Goleman, 1992; Gross, 1991; Vaughan, 1996); the struggle for civil rights (Naegle, 1993; Sack, 1993; Schmalz, 1993b; The Future, 1990) or the restriction of gay rights (Gross, 1992; Johnson, 1993); the anatomical idiosyncrasies of brains in gay men (Angier, 1991a, 1991b, 1992, 1993; Bailey and Pillard, 1991; Burr, 1993; Gelman, 1992; Henry, 1993; LeVey, 1991); the collective power of lesbians (Salholz et al., 1993); gay and lesbian content in school curriculums (Levy, 1992; Myers, 1992a, 1992b; Teaching about, 1992); gays and the Boy Scouts (Boy Scouts, 1992); the first gay comic book character (The comics, 1992); and, finally, the movement to end the ban on gays and lesbians in the military (Gay sailor, 1993; Gordon, 1993, Manegold, 1993, Schmitt, 1993a, 1993b, 1993c, Schmalz, 1993a). It seems that after years of being relegated to a whisper, the issues of gays and lesbians are now being dealt with openly and visibly.

The Internet and the World Wide Web have provided other very important sources of information that individuals can have access to within the confines of their own homes. The information superhighway has not only grown exponentially during the past several years, but has also provided a plethora of new information about a wide variety of topics pertaining to gay and lesbian persons. Although there are also inaccuracies on the Internet, one huge benefit for those seeking access to knowledge about gay men and lesbians is that the Web has a reach that exceeds geography. Consequently, persons in remote rural areas, as well as those in more urban centers potentially have equal access to information about and communication with gay men and lesbians around the world, whereas in the past such data was only to be found in urban environs. Albeit one must have access to a computer to make such connections, libraries and schools in many communities can provide individuals with such access.

A recent scan of relevant Web sites includes the following: The Gay and Lesbian Information site (http://www.ping.be/ping1678gay.); The Human Rights Campaign site (http://humanrights.org); The Gay and Lesbian Parents Coalition International (GLPCI) and Children of

Lesbians and Gays Everywhere (COLAGE) (http://www.qrd.org/
qrd/www/orgsglpci/home.htm); Parents and Friends of Lesbians and
Gays (PFLAG) (http://wwwcritpath.org/pflag-talk); The Straight
Spouses Network, a support group for men and women who are or
have been married to gay, lesbian, or bisexual spouses (http://www/
qrd.org/qrd/www/orgs/sssn/home.htm); Youth Action Line, a wonderful Web site for youth (http://www.youth.org/); the PERSON
Project Alerts Web site (http://www.youth.org/loco/PERSON proj-
ect/Alerts/list.html.), which maintains careful watch on a wide array
of issues that affect gay and lesbian persons. These are but a few
Web sites of the literally thousands that exist on the topic of gay
men and lesbians. The reader may find others through links with
any of the Web sites mentioned above, or may find additional sites
by using one of the numerous search engines (Yahoo, Webcrawler,
Lycos, Excite, and others) and by keying code words and phrases
such as gay, lesbian, bisexual, and sexual orientation.

It is, however, a trinity of historical phenomenons, including the
groundbreaking work of the late Dr. Evelyn Hooker (1957, 1967),
which presented the first rigorous scientific research to provide
indisputable evidence that homosexuality is not a mental illness; the
commencement of the Stonewall Rebellion of 1969 in New York
City, generally regarded as the nativity of the gay and lesbian liberation movement; and the elimination of homosexuality as a psychiatric disorder from the *Diagnostic and Statistical Manual of Mental
Disorders* (Third Edition) (DSM III) in 1973, that were the major
forces in conceptualizing Western society's views of gay and lesbian persons. In many significant ways, the advent of the AIDS
pandemic has been another defining event for gay men and lesbians.

Social work's history with gay men and lesbians can best be
described as an ambivalent relationship. Although the Delegate
Assembly of the National Association of Social Workers (1994a,
1994b) adopted a policy statement on gay issues in 1977 and reaf-
firmed its commitment to this statement in 1993, and updated its
code of ethics in 1994 and 1996 to emphasize its ban on discrimination based on sexual orientation, social work has generally lagged
behind other helping professionals in putting resources behind its
commitment.

Although the Council on Social Work Education (1992) revised its accreditation standards to require schools of social work to include foundation content related to lesbian and gay service needs and practice into the core course curriculum (see Humphreys, 1983; Newman, 1989), a motion was put forward at the council's 1996 annual meeting to waive this requirement for "certain religiously affiliated organizations." Such moves signal a reluctance on the part of the professional from allowing gay and lesbian persons full and equal access to being included in the curriculum (See Parr and Jones' 1996 recent "Point/Counterpoint" journal article for a more complete discussion on this topic).

Despite inclusive policies and accreditation mandates that call for nondiscriminatory professional practice, an inherent difficulty in separating personal attitudes from professional prerogatives with respect to homosexuality appears to have made service provision to this population a complex process. Homosexuality has historically been and continues to be a taboo subject for discussion even within most professional climates (Gochros, 1985, 1995; Mallon, 1992).

THE PROFESSIONAL LITERATURE

Although a plethora of professional literature has been published on and about gay men and lesbians in the *Journal of Homosexuality* and more recently in the *Journal of Gay and Lesbian Social Services,* the mainstream social work publications have lagged behind several of the other helping professions, most notably psychology, in recognizing the legitimacy of homosexuality in the professional literature.

If one were to look exclusively within the social work professional literature to develop a knowledge base of practice, one would find a very circumscribed discussion of gay and lesbian practice issues in the mainstream social work literature. The major social work journals have been slow to respond to and to publish articles that address the wide and diverse needs of gay men and lesbians. A recent review (Mallon, in review) of thirty years of coverage (1964-1993) of gay and lesbian issues in the social work literature of four major social work journals found that less than 1 percent (n = 38) of the total number of articles (n = 5,907) addressed the needs of this population. Unquestionably, there is a pressing need to provide information on and about lesbian and gay persons.

It is beyond the scope of this chapter to review the literature that delineates the knowledge requisite to achieve competent practice with gay men and lesbians; key components, however, are highlighted in Table 1.1.

TABLE 1.1. LITERATURE ON GAY MEN AND LESBIANS

Key Concepts and Terms

Appleby and Anastas, in press; Appleby and Anastas, 1992; Gochros, 1972; Hidalgo, Peterson, and Woodman, 1985; Moses and Hawkins, 1982; Schoenberg, Goldberg, and Shore, 1985

Understanding Heterocentrism and Homophobia: Theory, Manifestations and Implications for Practice

Albro and Tully, 1979; Berger and Kelly, 1981; DeCrescenzo, 1985; Dulaney and Kelly, 1982; Gramick, 1983; Reiter, 1991; Tievsky, 1988; Wisniewski and Toomey, 1987

Theories and Models of Gay and Lesbian Identity Formation and the Coming-Out Process

Chafetz, Sampson, Beck, and West, 1974; Chan, 1993; Espin, 1993; Folayan, 1992; Gock, 1992; Gutierrez, 1992; Hidalgo, 1995; Icard, 1985/1986; Lewis, 1984; Loiacano, 1993; Lukes and Land, 1990; Reiter, 1989; Sullivan, 1995; Tafoya, 1992; Williams, 1986, 1993

Bisexuality and Transgender Issues

Blumstein and Schwartz, 1977; Levine, 1978; Wicks, 1978

Social Work with Gay, Lesbian, and Bisexual Children and Adolescents

Cates, 1987; DeCrescenzo, 1995; Hunter and Schaecher, 1987, 1994; Jacobsen, 1988; Mallon, 1994; Malyon, 1981; Morrow, 1993; Needham, 1977; Savin-Williams 1989; Schneider, 1988, 1989; Schneider and Tremble, 1985; Sullivan and Schneider, 1987

Gays, Lesbians, and Bisexuals and Their Families

Auerback and Moser, 1987; deVine, 1983/1984; Gochros, 1989; Hall, 1978; Laird, 1983, 1996; Laird and Green, 1996; Lui and Chan, 1996; Mallon, in press b; Slater, 1995; Strommen, 1989; Wyers, 1987

Lesbian, Gay, and Bisexual Couples and Their Relationships

Berger, 1990; Decker, 1984; dePoy and Noble, 1992; Kurdek, 1994, 1995; Larson, 1982; McCandlish, 1985; Mc Whirter and Mattison, 1984; Peplau, 1993; Peplau and Amaro, 1982; Shernoff, 1995

Gays and Lesbians Raising Children: Adoption/Foster Parenting, Biological Parenting

Benkov, 1994; Bigner, 1996; Levy, 1992; Lewis, 1980; Mallon, 1992, in press c; Martin, 1993; Patterson, 1994; Ricketts and Achtenberg, 1990; Shernoff, 1996c

Lesbians and Gay Men in Midlife and Old Age

Berger, 1982, 1983, 1996; Berger and Kelly, 1981; Dorfman et al., 1995; Kehoe, 1988; Kimmel and Sang, 1995; Quam, 1997; Sang, 1993

Lesbian and Gay Health and Mental Health Concerns for the Social Work Practitioner

Baez, 1996; Friend, 1987; Huggins et al., 1991; Kus, 1995; Lloyd, 1992; Lloyd and Kuszelewicz, 1995; Loewenstein, 1980; Martin, 1991; Peterson, 1996; Renzetti and Miley, 1996; Scott and Shernoff, 1988; Shernoff, 1984; Woodman, 1992

Social Service Delivery: Programmatic and Administrative Issues

Anderson and Henderson, 1985; Ball, 1996; Beaton and Guild, 1976; Bernstein, 1977; Berger, 1977; Dulaney and Kelly, 1982; Gambe and Getzel, 1989; Gochros, 1975, 1985, 1992; Hartman, 1993; Icard, Schilling, El-Bassel, and Young, 1992; Icard and Traunstein, 1987; Lopez and Getzel, 1984; Morton, 1982; Potter and Darty, 1981; Rabin, et al., 1986; Tully and Albro, 1979

RESEARCH

Groups of people who have been oppressed and discriminated against are vulnerable to stereotyping, perpetuation of myths about them, and other forms of negative misinformation. The bedrock of such misinformation is heterocentrism, racism, ethnocentrism, ageism, sexism, or ableism, or all of these. Consequently, individuals who are members of oppressed groups may also believe or internalize these negative stereotypes about their group and thereby suffer what has been called a "dual oppression" (MacEachron, 1996, p. 20) from self and others. An important way to uncover stereotypic misinformation and oppressive myths is to provide evidence that validates the uniqueness of each individual. The amount of affirmative research, however, is not always congruent to the extent of societal oppression toward a group of people.

Both quantitative and qualitative methods of research, or a blend of the two, are important means toward generating knowledge that has a scientific basis. Naturalistic inquiry, which is the rigorous observation of phenomena that are important to social work practice, is particularly useful in cases where there has been limited conceptualization of an empirical nature. With its epistemological roots in anthropology, naturalistic research has increasingly been seen as an effective means of informing social work practice, particularly with gay men and lesbians.

Quantitative research has also found its place in allowing social workers to test sanctioned wisdom and to try new methods that may result in an improved outcome for clients. Group designs and single-system designs are probably the most common subtypes of experimental research. In the context of an emerging managed care environment, and as a means toward addressing issues of accountability, utilizing standardized outcome measures to test the veracity of clinical interventions with clients has increasingly become a significant aspect of practice (Bloom, Fischer, and Orme, 1995; Blythe, Tripodi, and Briar, 1994; Fischer and Corcoron, 1994; Hudson, 1985). Although only one standardized instrument could be found in the literature (Nurius and Hudson, 1988) to measure sexual orientation, there are two instruments (Hudson and Ricketts, 1980; Lumby, 1976) that were developed to measure homophobia.

In addition to monitoring practice effectiveness, quantitative methods have primarily been utilized by investigators who have sought to examine broad issues pertaining to the origin of sexual orientation (Acosta, 1975; Angier, 1991a, 1991b; 1992, 1993; Bailey and Pillard, 1991; Baranaga, 1991; Barringer, 1993; Bell, Weinberg, and Hammersmith, 1981; Burr, 1993a; Jay and Young, 1977; LeVey, 1991; Money, 1980; Money and Ehrhardt, 1972; Saghir, Robbins, and Walbian, 1973) and in the many attempts that have been made to quantify the population of gay men and lesbians (Janus and Janus, 1993; Kinsey, Pomeroy, and Martin, 1948;

Kinsey, Pomeroy, Martin, and Gebhard, 1953; National Opinion Research Center, 1989-1992; Rogers, 1993).

In a recent edited text, Tully (1996) and her colleagues (Jacobson, 1996; MacEachron, 1996; Woodman, Tully, and Barranti, 1996) focus on research issues with a lesbian population. Although the research that has focused on gay men has been slim in comparison to other groups, the research that has specifically focused on lesbians is even more sparse. Tully (1996) and her colleagues have provided researchers and scholars with an intelligent and comprehensive overview of the research issues that affect lesbians. This text can serve as a useful guide to those interested in examining research issues as a means toward developing practice knowledge about working with gay men and lesbians.

THEORETICAL AND CONCEPTUAL ANALYSES

Theories to guide practice or theoretical constructs that help one to better understand practice with a client system also offer explanations to guide practice. Understanding the process of gay and lesbian identity formation will undoubtedly enable the practitioner to carry out informed and sensitive intervention with clients and families struggling with issues of sexual orientation. However, practitioners must also be aware of the fact that it is not possible for them to utilize traditional developmental models taught in most human behavior and social environment sequences (Blos, 1979; Erikson, 1950; Marcia, 1980; Newman and Newman, 1987), which posit concepts of sex-role identifications that are concerned only with heterosexual development and presume heterosexual identity as an eventual outcome.

Since the 1960s, identity movements of oppressed people (e.g., women, people-of-color communities, people with disabilities, gay men and lesbians) have challenged both academia and the larger society by exposing the extent to which they have been neglected by prevailing theoretical models (Domenici and Lesser, 1995). By exposing the biases behind paradigms that were previously considered objective, these voices have revealed the extent to which all epistemology is discourse specific (Domenici and Lesser, 1995). Dominant groups have constructed narratives of oppressed people that strengthened their own needs, values, interests, and self-esteem. Utilizing traditional approaches, which view homosexuality from a developmentally pejorative perspective, does not assist or prepare the practitioner to work competently with gay or lesbian persons.

Berger, who has written broadly (1977, 1982, 1983, 1990, 1996) about social work practice with gay and lesbian persons, offered two models for working with persons who identify as gay or lesbian: an advocate model (1977) and a definitional model (1983). Falco (1991), Garnets et al., (1991), and Morin (1991) have also presented affirmative models of therapy with lesbians and gay men. Viewing homosexuality through a lens of biculturality, Lukes and Lands (1990) proposed a model of practice that linked cultural issues with issues of one's identity. More recently, Slater's (1995) work also provided an affirming framework for working lesbian clients within the context of a family life cycle.

Unlike their counterparts in the heterosexual majority, gay men and lesbians experience a social condition that is attributable to their gay or lesbian sexual orientation-oppression. Oppression, notes Pharr (1988), cannot be viewed in isolation because its various dimensions—sexism, racism, homophobia, classism, anti-Semitism, and ableism,—are interconnected by a common origin-economic power and control. Backed by institutional power, economic power, and both institutional and individual violence, this trinity of elements acts as the "standard of rightness and often righteousness wherein all others are judged in relation to it."

There are many ways that norms are enforced both by individuals and institutions. One way to view persons who fall outside the "norm" is to label such individuals as "the other." It is easy to discriminate against—view as deviant, marginal, or inferior—such groups that are not part of the mainstream. Those who are classified as such become part of an invisible minority, a group whose achievements are kept hidden and unknown from those in the dominant culture. Stereotyping, blaming the victim, and distortion of reality can even lead the person to feeling as though they deserve the oppression that they experience. This process is called internalized homophobia. Other elements of oppression include isolation, passing as heterosexual, self-hatred, underachievement or overachievement, substance abuse, problems with relationships, and a variety of other mental health matters.

Violence, as suggested by Hanson (1996), Herek, (1990) Hunter (1990), and Pharr (1988) is also seen as a theoretical construct in the lives of gay and lesbian persons. The threat of violence toward gay men and women who step out of line is made all the more powerful by the fact that they do not have to do anything to receive the violence. It is their lives alone that precipitate such action. Therefore, gay men and lesbians always have a sense of safety that is fragile and tenuous, and they may never feel completely secure. Social workers who are unfamiliar with gay and lesbians persons may view such conditions as a pathology in need of treatment, but for the gay or lesbian person such insecurity is an adaptive strategy for living within in a hostile environment (Germain and Gitterman, 1996).

SELF-AWARENESS

Many students entering the world of social work think that they are open minded, and while many may have a genuine desire to help others, some have not delved inside of themselves to assess the roles that power, privilege, and influence have played in their own lives.

As social work is a values-based profession (McGowan, 1995), we are ethically obligated to address these issues and to work toward increasing the levels of competence and awareness within both students entering the profession and colleagues who continue to make contributions. Although the professional literature has begun to address these areas, as professionals we also must focus on the issue of self-awareness.

The consequence of not considering theoretical analyses and concepts that are heterocentric is that many heterosexual social workers believe that if they avoid society's fear and loathing of gay men and lesbians then it is all that they need to do to work effectively with gay men and lesbian clients. While most social workers have "politically correct" ideas about gay men and lesbians, many professionals have not always had the opportunity to deal with the deeper prejudices and heterosexual privileges that they, themselves, possess. Since most professionals continue to have an inadequate knowledge base about the real lives of gay men and lesbians, this causes them to be in many cases more homoignorant than homophobic.

Many gay and lesbian persons believe that heterosexually oriented social workers still harbor the heterocentric assumption that it is less than normal or less preferable to be gay or lesbian. Some social workers, particularly those from a more psychoanalytically oriented perspective, believe that somewhere in the gay or lesbian person's system you can find the roots or the cause of homosexuality and that it secretly has something to do with family dysfunction (Markowitz, 1991b, p. 28).

These are complex issues that need to be addressed within the overall context of diversity and yet at the same time from a specific gay and lesbian perspective. Moral, religious, and cultural biases still run deep in many students preparing for practice and in professionals who currently practice. Although there are no simple solutions to helping individuals overcome their biases, beginning an honest dialogue and providing students with accurate and appropriate information about gay men and lesbians is an important place to start.

KNOWLEDGE DERIVED FROM THE INDIVIDUAL CASE

Information provided by the case itself is the final means toward the generation of knowledge about gay and lesbian persons that will be discussed in this chapter. The client within the individual, couple, family, community, or organizational system, and the environmental context within which they live provide a great deal of information which is specific to the case and which can guide practice. Listening to what clients say and observing what they do from initial engagement through assessment, intervention, and termination can provide crucial information.

Eda Goldstein (1995), in her chapter on ego-oriented intervention with diverse and oppressed populations, speaks to this type of knowledge, as she succinctly points out,

> Homosexuality is not a psychiatric illness nor does its presence in men and women mean that they are suffering from a

disease that needs to be cured or that they are showing psychological maladjustment or some type of personality pathology. (p. 249)

Although some gay men and lesbians present concerns that relate specifically to issues of sexual orientation, many of which will be discussed in Shernoff and Steinhorn's essays in this collection, these individuals "usually seek help for a range of issues that have little to do with their sexual orientation per se or are related to it in an indirect way" (Goldstein, 1995, p. 249). Like their heterosexual counterparts, gay and lesbian persons seek help from social work practitioners to deal with a wide array of problems in living.

A critical aspect of intervening with a client who identifies as gay, lesbian, or bisexual is for practitioners to have a firm understanding of the client's identity formation, or what is more commonly known as the coming-out process (Cass, 1979, 1983/1984, 1984; Coleman, 1981, 1987; DeMonteflores and Schultz, 1978; Troiden, 1979, 1988, 1989). Although the adolescent and young adult (Hetrick and Martin, 1987) periods of development are extremely important for gay identity development, the coming out process can occur at any point in the life course, particularly for women (Cass, 1996; Falco, 1991; Gramick, 1984; Ponse, 1980; Sophie, 1985-1986), and may extend over many years.

The practitioner who is sensitive and affirming in his or her work with gay and lesbian persons needs to have a complete understanding of the psychological, behavioral, affectional, attitudinal, and internal sense of "goodness of fit" as the features of each of the stages of coming out and should direct their interventions accordingly. A lack of familiarity with this process will cause the practitioner to misinterpret the client's reactions and to miss opportunities to assist the client in moving forward in the process of developing a comfort with their own identity.

Practitioners need to be aware that certain conditions may be intensified, if not caused, by oppression and stigmatization to which gay men and lesbians may have been exposed in their development and which they may continue to experience as adults. For example, although the coming-out process has been conceptualized as a positive developmental step toward healthfulness, the societal or familial response to an individual's disclosure may be less than constructive. On the other hand, the psychological consequences of hiding or passing (Berger, 1990; Cain, 1991a, 1991b) are great and often contribute to conflict experienced on individual, interpersonal, and group levels.

Social work practitioners need to be sensitive to the particular needs and concerns of the gay or lesbian person and must also appreciate that the client's membership in a stigmatized and oppressed group (Goffman, 1963) has shaped his or her identity and may play a role in the presenting problem they may or may not bring to their initial session. Whether or not the presenting problem is related to the client's sexual orientation, the practitioner who intervenes with the client must be well acquainted with the issues and features of gay or lesbian life, develop an expertise in working with the population, and acquire a knowledge of the community resources that exist to help this client. It is also important to recognize that there is as much diversity in the gay and lesbian community as in all other communities, and therefore, there is no one type of gay or lesbian individual.

Although Western society has made some positive steps in altering negative attitudes toward gay men and lesbians, practitioners, in working with individuals, must be aware of the presence of internalized homophobia (Malyon, 1982; Martin, 1982) and a client's own refrain from reinforcing it through his or her own bias and stereotypes. Isolation is another problem that frequently arises as a result of the stigma associated with a gay or lesbian identity. Practitioners need to be knowledgeable about resources that exist in the community and, if necessary, need to support the client by going with him or her to visit these resources. The development of social support networks through involvement in such programs can be an important task for the client and practitioner to work on together.

Despite the mitigating effects of oppression, stigma, and discrimination, gay men and lesbians are a resilient and resourceful group of people who possess many strengths (Berger, 1990; Mallon, in press a). Utilizing a strength's perspective of practice (Cowger, 1994; DeJong and Miller, 1995) is also an important strategy in not only gaining knowledge about clients, but also as a step toward affirming and acknowledging the dignity and worth of individuals.

Subsequent chapters in this book will focus on exploring social work practice with gay and lesbian persons from the perspectives of several client systems: individuals, groups, couples, families, communities, and organizations.

CONCLUSION

Although the vast majority of gay men and lesbians are healthy, resilient, and hardy individuals who do not seek social work intervention, some gay and lesbian persons have been or will be clients in the agencies where social workers practice. Training social workers in our MSW programs and in our agencies is not only a requirement of Council on Social Work Education, which is affirmed by the National Association of Social Workers, but is also an ethical responsibility of the profession. Cultivating a knowledge base of practice to prepare students and practitioners to work more competently and effectively with gay men and lesbians is an essential element of good practice and needs to be integrated into a foundation level curriculum in meaningful and conscientious ways.

REFERENCES

Acosta, F. X. (1975). Etiology and treatment of homosexuality: A review. *Archives of Sexual Behavior, 4,* 9-29.

Albro, J. C. and Tully, C. (1979). A study of lesbian lifestyles in the homosexual micro-culture and the heterosexual macro-culture. *Journal of Homosexuality, 4*(4), 331-344.

American Psychiatric Association. (1975). *Diagnostic and Statistical Manual of Mental Disorders* (third edition) (DSM III.) Washington, DC: American Psychiatric Association.

Anderson, S. and Henderson, D. (1985). Working with lesbian alcoholics. *Social Casework, 30*(6), 518-526.

Angier, N. (1991a September 1). Zone of brain linked to men's sexual orientation. *The New York Times,* p. A1.

Angier, N. (1991b September 7). The biology of what it means to be gay. *The New York Times,* p. D1.

Angier, N. (1992 August 1). Researchers find a second anatomical idiosyncrasy in brains of homosexual men. *The New York Times,* p. B1.

Angier, N. (1993 March 12). Study suggests genes sway lesbians' sexual orientation. *The New York Times,* p. A11.

Appleby, G. and Anastas, J. (1992). Social work practice with lesbians and gays. In A. Morales and B. Sheafor (Eds.), *Social work: A profession with many faces.* (pp. 347-381). New York: Allyn and Bacon.

Appleby, G. and Anastas, J. (in press.) *Not just a passing phase.* New York: Columbia University Press.

Auerback, S. and Moser, C. (1987). Groups for the wives of gay and bisexual men. *Social Work, 32*(4), 321-325.

Baez, E. (1996). Spirituality and the gay Latino client. In M. Shernoff (Ed.), *Human services for gay people: Clinical and community practice* (pp. 69-82). Binghamton, NY: Harrington Park Press.

Bailey, M. and Pillard, R. (1991 August 17). Are some people born gay? *The New York Times,* p. A33.

Ball, S. (1996). HIV-negative men: Individual and community social service needs. In M. Shernoff (Ed.), *Human services for gay people: Clinical and community practice* (pp. 25-40). Binghamton, NY: Harrington Park Press.

Baranaga, M. (1991, August 31). Is homosexuality biological? *Science, 252*(5023), p. 945-958.

Barringer, F. (1993 April 15). Sex survey of American men finds 1% are gay. *The New York Times,* p. A1.

Beaton, S. and Guild, N. (1976). Treatment for gay problem drinkers. *Social Casework, 57,* 302-308.

Bell, A. P., Weinberg, M. S., and Hammersmith, S. K. (1981). *Sexual preference: Its development in men and women.* Bloomington: University of Indiana Press.

Benkov, L. (1994). *Reinventing the family: The emerging story of lesbian and gay parents.* New York: Crown Publishers.

Bennet, J. (1993 January 11). Registry for gay couples holds benefits and risks. *The New York Times,* p. B3.

Berger, R. M. (1977). An advocate model for intervention with homosexuals. *Social Work, 22*(4), 280-283.

Berger, R. M. (1982). The unseen minority: Older gays and lesbians. *Social Work, 27*(3), 236-242.

Berger, R. M. (1983). What is a homosexual? A definitional model. *Social Work, 28*(2), 132-135.

Berger, R.M. (1990). Passing: Impact on the quality of same-sex couple relationships. *Social Work, 35,* 328-332.

Berger, R. M. (1996). *Gay and gray* (second edition). Boston: Alyson Publications.

Berger, R. M. and Kelly, J. J. (1981). Do social work agencies discriminate against homosexual job applicants? *Social Work, 26*(3), 193-198.

Bernstein, B.E. (1977). Legal and social interface in counseling homosexual clients. *Social Casework, 58*(1), 36-40.

Bigner, J. (1996). Working with gay fathers. In J. Laird and R-J. Green (Eds.), *Lesbians and gays in couples and families: A handbook for therapists* (pp. 370-403). San Francisco: Jossey-Bass Publishers.

Bloom, M., Fischer, J., and Orme, J. G. (1995). *Evaluating practice: Guidelines for the accountable professional* (second edition). Needham Heights, MA: Allyn and Bacon.

Blos, P. (1979). *The adolescent passage: Development issues.* New York: International Universities Press.

Blumstein, P. W. and Schwartz, P. (1977). Bisexuality: Some social psychological issues. *Journal of Social Issues, 33*(2), 30-45.

Blythe, B., Tripodi, T., and Briar, S. (1994). *Direct practice research in human service agencies.* New York: Columbia University Press.

Boys Scouts to allow homosexuals in the new program. (1992 August 22). *The New York Times,* p. A15.

Burr, C. (1993 March). Homosexuality and biology. *The Atlantic Monthly, 271*(3), 47-65.

Cain, R. (1991a). Relational contexts and information management among gay men. *Families in Society, 72*(6), 344-352.

Cain, R. (1991b). Stigma management and gay identity development. *Social Work, 36*(1), 67-73.

Cain, R. (1996). Heterosexism and disclosure in the social work classroom. *Journal of Social Work Education, 32*(1), 65-76.

Cass, V. C. (1979). Homosexual identity formation: A theoretical model. *Journal of Homosexuality, 4,* 219-235.

Cass, V. C. (1983/1984). Homosexual identity: A concept in need of a definition. *Journal of Homosexuality, 9*(2/3), 105-126.

Cass, V. C. (1984). Homosexual identity formation: Testing a theoretical model. *Journal of Sex Research, 20,* 143-167.

Cass, V. C. (1996 July 16). Personal interview.

Cates, J.A. (1987). Adolescent sexuality: Gay and lesbian issues. *Child Welfare League of America, 66,* 353-363.

Chafetz, J. S., Sampson, P., Beck, P., and West, J. (1974). A study of homosexual women. *Social Work, 19*(6), 714-723.

Chan, C. (1993). Issues of identity development among Asian American lesbians and gay men. In L.D. Garnets and D. G. Kimmel (Eds.), *Psychological perspectives on lesbian and gay male experiences* (pp. 376-388). New York: Columbia University Press.

Coleman, E. (1981). Developmental stages of the coming out process. *Journal of Homosexuality, 7*(2/3), 31-43.

Coleman, E. (1987). Assessment of sexual orientation. *Journal of Homosexuality, 13*(4), 9-23.

The comics break new ground again. (1992 January 24). *The New York Times,* p. A33.

Council on Social Work Education. (1992). *Curriculum policy statement for master's degree programs in social work education.* Alexandria, VA: Council on Social Work Education.

Cowger, C. D. (1994). Assessing client strengths: Clinical assessment for client empowerment. *Social Work, 39*(3), 262-268.

Decker, B. (1984). Counseling gay and lesbian couples. In R. Schoenberg and R. Goldberg (Eds.), *Homosexuality and social work* (pp. 39-52). Binghamton, NY: Harrington Park Press.

DeCrescenzo, T. (1985). Homophobia: A study of attitudes of mental health professionals towards homosexuality. In R. Schoenberg, R. Goldberg, and D. Shore (Eds.), *With compassion towards some: Homosexuality and social work in America* (pp. 115-136). Binghamton, NY: Harrington Park Press.

DeCrescenzo, T. (Ed.). (1995). *Helping gay and lesbian youth: New policies, new programs, new practices.* Binghamton, NY: The Haworth Press.

DeJong, P. and Miller, S. D. (1995). How to interview for client strength. *Social Work, 40*(6), 729-736.

DeMonteflores, C. and Schultz, S. J. (1978). Coming out: Similarities and differences for lesbians and gay men. *Journal of Social Issues, 34*(3), 59-72.

dePoy, E. and Noble, S. (1992). The structure of lesbian relationships in response to oppression. *Affilia, 7*(4), 49-64.

deVine, J. L. (1983/1984). A systemic inspection of affectional preference orientation and family of origin. *Journal of Social Work and Human Sexuality, 2* (2/3), 9-17.

Domenici, T. and Lesser, R.C. (Eds). (1995). *Disorienting sexuality: Psychoanalytic reappraisals of sexual identities.* New York: Routledge.

Dorfman, R., Walters, K., Burke, P., Hardin, L., Karanik, T., Raphael, J., and Silverstein, E. (1995). Old, sad, and alone: The myth of the aging homosexual. *Journal of Gerontological Social Work, 24*(1/2), 29-44.

Dulaney, D. D. and Kelly, J. J. (1982). Improving services to gay and lesbian clients. *Social Work, 27*(2), 178-183.

English, M. (1996). Transgenerational homophobia in the family: A personal narrative. In J. Laird and R-J. Green (Eds.), *Lesbians and gays in couples and families: A handbook for therapists* (pp. 15-27). San Francisco: Jossey-Bass Publishers.

Erikson, E. (1950). *Childhood and society.* New York: W.W. Norton and Co.

Espin, O. (1993). Issues of identity in the psychology of Latina lesbians. In L. D. Garnets and D. G. Kimmel (Eds.), *Psychological perspectives on lesbian and gay male experiences* (pp. 348-363). New York: Columbia University Press.

Falco, K. L. (1991). *Psychotherapy with lesbian clients.* New York: Brunner/Mazel.

Fischer, J. and Corcoron, K. (1994). *Measures for clinical practice: A sourcebook,* second edition (Volumes 1 and 2). New York: The Free Press.

Folayan, A. (1992). African-American issues: The soul of it. In B. Berzon (Ed.), *Positively gay* (pp. 235-239). Berkeley, CA: Celestial Arts.

Friend, R. (1987). The individual and social psychology of aging: Clinical implications for lesbians and gay men. *Journal of Homosexuality, 14*(1/2), 25-44.

The future of gay America. (1990 March 12). *Newsweek,* 20-27.

Gambe, R. and Getzel, G. S. (1989). Group work with gay men with AIDS. *Social Casework, 70*(3), 172-179.

Garnets, L., Hancock, K. A., Cochran, S. D., Goodchilds, J., and Peplau, L. A. (1991). Issues in psychotherapy with lesbians and gay men: A survey of psychologists. *American Psychologist, 46,* 964-972.

Gartrell, N. K. (1994). Boundaries in lesbian therapist-client relationships. In B. Greene and G. M. Herek (Eds.), *Lesbian and gay psychology: Theory, research, and clinical applications* (pp. 98-117). Thousand Oaks, CA: Sage Publications.

Gay adoption cases go to appeals court. (1993 April 18). *The New York Times,* p. A25.

Gay sailor tells of a "living hell." (1993 March 8). *The New York Times,* p. A15.

Gelman, D. (1992 February 24). Born or bred? *Newsweek,* 46-53.

Germain, C. B. (1991). *Human behavior and the social environment.* New York: Columbia University Press.

Germain, C. B. and Gitterman, A. (1996). *The life model of social work practice,* second edition. New York: Columbia University Press.

Gochros, H. (1972). The sexually oppressed. *Social Work, 17,* 16-23.

Gochros, H. (1975). Teaching more or less straight social work students to be helpful to more or less gay people. *The Homosexual Counseling Journal, 2*(2), 24-31.

Gochros, H. (1992). The sexuality of gay men with HIV infection. *Social Work, 37*(2), 105-109.

Gochros, H. (1995). Sex, AIDS, social work and me. *Reflections, 1*(2), 37-43.

Gochros, H. L. (1985). Teaching social workers to meet the needs of the homosexually oriented. In R. Schoenberg, R. Goldberg, and D. Shore (Eds.), *With compassion towards some: Homosexuality and social work in America* (pp. 137-156). Binghamton, NY: Harrington Park Press.

Gochros, J. (1989). *When husbands come out of the closet.* Binghamton, NY: The Haworth Press.

Gock, T. (1992). Asian-Pacific islander issues: Identity integration and pride. In B. Berzon (Ed.), *Positively gay* (pp. 247-252). Berkeley, CA: Celestial Arts.

Goffman, E. (1963). *Stigma: Notes of the management of a spoiled identity.* Englewood Cliffs, NJ: Prentice-Hall.

Goldstein, E. (1995). *Ego psychology and social work practice,* second edition. New York: The Free Press.

Goleman, D. (1992 December 2). Studies find no disadvantage in growing up in a gay home. *The New York Times,* p. C14.

Gordon, M. R. (1993 March 30). Senate hearings open on homosexuals in military. *The New York Times,* p. A18.

Gramick, J. (1983). Homophobia: A new challenge. *Social Work, 28*(2), 137-141.

Gramick, J. (1984). Developing a lesbian identity. In T. Darty and S. Potter (Eds.), *Women identified women* (pp. 31-44). Palo Alto, CA: Mayfield.

Greene, B. (1994). Lesbian and gay sexual orientations: Implications for clinical training, practice and research. In B. Greene and G. M. Herek (Eds.), *Lesbian and gay psychology: Theory, research, and clinical applications* (pp. 1-24). Thousand Oaks, CA: Sage Publications.

Greene, R. (1994) *Human behavior theory: A diversity framework.* Hawthorne, NY: Aldine de Gruyter.

Gross, J. (1991 February 11). New challenges of youth: Growing up in a gay home. *The New York Times,* p. A1.

Gross, J. (1992 September 26). In reversal, California governor signs a bill extending gay rights. *The New York Times,* p. A1.

Gutierrez, E. (1992). Latino issues: Gay and lesbian Latinos claiming La Raza. In B. Berzon (Ed.), *Positively gay* (pp. 247-252). Berkeley, CA: Celestial Arts.

Hall, M. (1978). Lesbian families: Cultural and clinical issues. *Social Work, 23*(5), 31-35.

Hanson, B. (1996). The violence we face as lesbians and gay men: The landscape both outside and inside our communities. In M. Shernoff (Ed.), *Human services for gay people: Clinical and community practice* (pp. 95-114). Binghamton, NY: Harrington Park Press.

Hartman, A. (1992). In search of subjugated knowledge. *Social Work, 37,* 483-484.

Hartman, A. (1993). Out of the closet: Revolution and backlash. *Social Work, 38*(3), 245-246, 360.

Henry, W. A. (1993 July 26). Born gay? *Newsweek,* p. 36-39.

Herek, G. M. (1990). The context of anti-gay violence: Notes on cultural psychological heterosexism. *Journal of Interpersonal Violence, 5*(3), 316-333.

Hetrick, E. and Martin, A. D. (1987). Developmental issues and their resolution for gay and lesbian adolescents. *Journal of Homosexuality, 13*(4), 25-43.

Hidalgo, H. (Ed.). (1995). Lesbians of color: Social and human services. [Special Issue]. *Journal of Gay and Lesbian Social Services, 3*(2).

Hidalgo, H., Peterson, T. L., and Woodman, N. J. (Eds.). (1985). *Lesbian and gay issues: A resource manual for social workers.* Silver Springs, MD: National Association of Social Workers.

Hooker, E. (1957). The adjustment of the male overt homosexual. *Journal of Projective Techniques, 21,* 18-31.

Hooker, E. (1967). The homosexual community. In Gagnon, J. and Simon, W. (Eds.), *Sexual deviance* (pp. 380-392). New York: Harper and Row.

Hudson, W. W. (1985). The clinical assessment system [Computer program]. Tempe, AZ: University of Arizona School of Social Work.

Hudson, W. W. and Ricketts, W. A. (1980). A strategy for measurement of homophobia. *Journal of Homosexuality, 5,* 357-371.

Humphreys, G. E. (1983). Inclusion of content on homosexuality in the social work curriculum. *Journal of Social Work Education, 19*(1), 55-60.

Hunter, J. (1990). Violence against lesbian and gay male youths. *Journal of Interpersonal Violence, 5*(3), 295-300.

Hunter, J. and Schaecher, R. (1987). Stresses on lesbian and gay adolescents in schools. *Social Work in Education* (Spring), 180-188.

Hunter, J. and Schaecher, R. (1994). AIDS prevention for lesbian, gay, and bisexual adolescents. *Families and Society, 75*(6), 93-99.

Icard, L. (1985/1986). Black gay men and conflicting social identities: Sexual orientation versus racial identity. *Journal of Social Work and Human Sexuality, 4*(1-2), 83-93.

Icard, L. D., Schilling, R. F., El-Bassel, N., and Young, D. (1992). Preventing AIDS among black gay men and black gay and heterosexual male intravenous drug users. *Social Work, 37*(5), 440-445.

Icard, L. D. and Traunstein, D. M. (1987). Black, gay, alcoholic men: Their character and treatment. *Social Casework, 68*(5), 267-272.

Jacobsen. E. E. (1988). Lesbian and gay adolescents: A social work approach. *Social Worker/Le Travailler Social, 56*(2), 65-67.

Jacobson, S. (1996). Methodological research issues in research on older lesbians. In C. Tully (Ed.), *Lesbian social services: Research issues* (pp. 43-56). Binghamton, NY: The Haworth Press.

Janus, S. S. and Janus, C. L. (1993). *The Janus report on sexual behavior.* New York: John Wiley and Sons.

Jay, K. and Young, A. (1977). *The gay report: Lesbians and gay men speak out about their sexual experiences and lifestyles.* New York: Summit.

Johnson, D. (1993 January 16). A ban on gay-rights laws is put on hold in Colorado. *The New York Times,* p. A16.

Judge lets gay partner adopt child: Companion of mother becomes foster parent (1992 January 31). *The New York Times,* p. B1.

Kaplan, L. and Girard, J. L. (1994). *Strengthening high-risk families: A handbook for practitioners.* New York: Lexington Books.

Kehoe, M. (1988). *Lesbians over 60 speak for themselves.* Binghamton, NY: Harrington Park Press.

Kimmel, D. C. and Sang, B. E. (1995). Lesbians and gay men in midlife. In A. R. D'Augelli and C. J. Patterson (Eds.), *Gay, lesbian, and bisexual identities over the lifespan* (pp. 190-214). Oxford: Oxford University Press.

Kinsey, A. C., Pomeroy, W. B., and Martin, C. E. (1948). *Sexual behavior in the human male.* Philadelphia: W. B. Saunders.

Kinsey, A. C., Pomeroy, W. B., Martin, C. E., and Geghard, P. H. (1953). *Sexual behavior in the human female.* Philadelphia: W.B. Saunders.

Kurdek, L. A. (Ed.). (1994). Social services for gay and lesbian couples. [Special Issue]. *Journal of gay and lesbian Social Services, 1*(2).

Kurdek, L. A. (1995). Lesbian and gay couples. In A. R. D'Augelli and C. J. Patterson (Eds.), *Gay, lesbian, and bisexual identities over the lifespan* (pp. 243-261). Oxford: Oxford University Press.

Kus, R. J. (Ed.). (1995). Addition and recovery in gay and lesbian persons. [Special Issue]. *Journal of Gay and Lesbian Social Services, 2*(1).

Laird, J. (1983). Lesbian and gay families. In F. Walsh (Ed.), *Normal family processes,* fourth edition (pp. 282-328). New York: Guilford Press.

Laird, J. (1996). Invisible ties: Lesbians and their families of origin. In J. Laird and R-J. Green (Eds.), *Lesbians and gays in couples and families: A handbook for therapists* (pp. 89-122). San Francisco: Jossey-Bass Publishers.

Laird, J. and Green, R-J. (Eds.). (1996). *Lesbians and gays in couples and families*. San Francisco: Jossey-Bass Publishers.

Larson, P. C. (1982). Gay male relationships. In W. Paul, J.D. Weinrich, J.C. Gonsiorek, and M. E. Hotvedt (Eds.), *Homosexuality: Social, psychological and biological issues* (pp. 219-232). Beverly Hills, CA: Sage Press.

LeVey, S. (1991 August 31). A difference in hypothalamic structure between heterosexual and homosexual men. *Science, 253* (5023), pp. 1034-1037.

Levine, C.O. (1978). Social work with transsexuals. *Social Casework, 59*(3), 167-174.

Levy, E. F. (1992). Strengthening the coping resources of lesbian families. *Families in Society, 73*(1), 23-31.

Lewis, K. G. (1980). Children of lesbians: Their point of view. *Social Work, 25*(3), 198-203.

Lewis, L. A. (1984). The coming-out process for lesbians: Integrating a stable identity. *Social Work, 29*(5), 464-469.

Lloyd, G. A. (1992). Contextual and clinical issues in providing services to gay men. In H. Land (Ed.), *AIDS: A complete guide to psychosocial intervention* (pp. 91-105). Milwaukee: Family Services of America.

Lloyd, G. A. and Kuszelewicz, M. A. (Eds.). (1995). HIV disease: Lesbians, gays and the social services. [Special Issue]. *Journal of Gay and Lesbian Social Services, 2*(3/4).

Loewenstein, S. F. (1980). Understanding lesbian women. *Social Casework, 61*(1), 29-38.

Loiacano, D. (1993). Gay identity issues among black Americans: Racism, homophobia and the need for validation. In L. D. Garnets and D. G. Kimmel (Eds.), *Psychological perspectives on lesbian and gay male experiences* (pp. 364-375). New York: Columbia University Press.

Lopez, D. J. and Getzel, G. S. (1984). Helping gay AIDS patients in crisis. *Social Casework, 65*(7), 387-394.

Lui, P. and Chan, C. S. (1996). Lesbian, gay, and bisexual Asian-Americans and their families. In J. Laird and R-J. Green (Eds.), *Lesbians and gays in couples and families: A handbook for therapists* (pp. 137-152). San Francisco: Jossey-Bass Publishers.

Lukes, C. A. and Lands, H. (1990). Biculturality and homosexuality. *Social Work, 35*(2), 155-161.

Lumby, M. E. (1976). Homophobia: The quest for a valid scale. *The Journal of Homosexuality, 2*(1), 39-47.

MacEachron, A. E. (1996). Potential use of single-system design for evaluating affirmative psychotherapy with lesbian women and gay men. In C. Tully (Ed.), *Lesbian social services: Research issues* (pp. 19-28). Binghamton, NY: The Haworth Press.

MacPike, L. (Ed.). (1989). *There's something I've been meaning to tell you*. Tallahassee, FL: The Naiad Press.

Mallon, G. P. (1992). Gay and no place to go: Serving the needs of gay and lesbian youth in out-of-home care settings. *Child Welfare, 71*(6), 547-557.

Mallon, G. P. (1994). Counseling strategies with gay and lesbian youth. In T. DeCrescenzo (Ed.), *Helping gay and lesbian youth: New policies, new programs, new practices* (pp. 75-91). Binghamton, NY: The Haworth Press.

Mallon, G. P. (in press a). Gay, lesbian and bisexual childhood and adolescent development: An ecological perspective. In G. Appleby and J. Anastas (Eds.), *Not just a passing phase: Social work with gay, lesbian and bisexual persons.* New York: Columbia University Press.

Mallon, G. P. (in press b). Gay and lesbian adolescents and their families. In T. DeCrescenzo (Ed.), *Gay and lesbian youth.* Binghamton, NY: The Haworth Press.

Mallon, G. P. (in press c). *We don't exactly get the welcome wagon: The experience of gay and lesbian adolescents in North America's child welfare system.* New York: Columbia University Press.

Mallon, G. P. (in review). Coverage of gay and lesbian issues in four social work journals—1969-1993. *Social Work Research.*

Malyon, A. K. (1981). The homosexual adolescent: Developmental issues and social bias. *Child Welfare League of America, 60*(5), 321-330.

Malyon, A. K. (1982). Psychotherapeutic implications of internalized homophobia in gay men. *Journal of Homosexuality, 7*(2/3), 59-69.

Manegold, C. S. (1993 April 18). Playing it straight in the military: The odd place of homosexuality in the military. *The New York Times,* p. 4-1.

Marcia, J. E. (1980). Identity in adolescence. In J. Adelson (Ed.), *Handbook of adolescent psychiatry* (pp.159-187). New York: John Wiley & Sons.

Markowitz, L. (1991a). You can go home again. *The Family Therapy Networker, 2,* 55-60.

Markowitz, L. (1991b). Homosexuality: Are we still in the dark? *The Family Therapy Networker, 2,* 27-35.

Martin, A. (1991). Power of empathic relationships: Bereavement therapy with a lesbian widow. In C. Silverstein, (Ed.), *Gays, lesbians, and their therapists* (pp.172-186). New York: W.W. Norton and Co.

Martin, A. (1993). *The lesbian and gay parenting handbook: Creating and raising our families.* New York: Harper Perennial.

Martin, A. D. (1982). Learning to hide: The socialization of the gay adolescent. In S. C. Feinstein, J. G. Looney, A. Schartzberg, and A. Sorosky (Eds.), *Adolescent psychiatry: Developmental and clinical studies* (Volume 10) (pp. 52-65). Chicago: University of Chicago Press.

Mattaini, M. (1995). Knowledge for practice. In C. Meyer and M. Mattaini (Eds.), *Foundations of social work practice* (pp. 59-85). Washington, DC: National Association of Social Workers.

McCandlish, B. M. (1985). Therapeutic issues with lesbian couples. In J.C. Gonsiorek (Ed.), *A guide to psychotherapy with gay and lesbian clients,* (pp.71-78). Binghamton, NY: Harrington Park Press.

McGowan, B. (1995, October 16). Personal communication.

McWhirter, D. P. and Mattison, A. M. (1984). *The male couple: How relationships develop.* Engelwood Cliff, NJ: Prentice-Hall.

Meyer, C. (1982). Issues in clinical social work: In search of a consensus. In P. Carloff (Ed.), *Treatment formulations and clinical social work* (pp. 19-26). Silver Spring, MD: National Association of Social Workers.

Money, J. (1980). Genetic and chromosomal aspects of homosexual etiology. In J. Marmor (Ed.), *Homosexual behavior: A modern appraisal* (pp. 233-249). New York: Basic Books.

Money, J. and Ehrhardt, A. A. (1972). *Man and woman, boy and girl: The differentiation and dimorphism of gender identity from conception to maturity.* Baltimore: Johns Hopkins University Press.

Morin, S. F. (1991). Removing the stigma: Lesbian and gay affirmative counseling. *The counseling psychologist, 19,* 245-247.

Morrow, D. F. (1993). Social work with gay and lesbian adolescents. *Social Work, 38*(6), 655-660.

Morton, D. R. (1983). Strategies in probation: Treating gay offenders. *Social Casework, 63*(6), 33-38.

Moses, A. E. and Hawkins, R. D. (1982). *Counseling lesbian women and gay men.* St. Louis: Mosby.

Muzio, C. (1996). Lesbians choosing children: Creating families, creating narratives. In J. Laird and R-J. Green (Eds.), *Lesbians and gays in couples and families: A handbook for therapists* (pp. 358-369). San Francisco: Jossey-Bass Publishers.

Naegle, W. (1993 May 8). Group rights advocates fan flames of bias. *The New York Times,* p. A19.

National Association of Social Workers. (1994a). Lesbian and gay issues. In National Association of Social Workers (Eds.), *Social work speaks* (pp. 162-165). Washington, DC: National Association of Social Workers (NASW).

National Association of Social Workers. (1994b). *NASW Code of Ethics.* Washington, DC: NASW.

National Opinion Research Center. (1989-1992). *General social survey.* University of Chicago: Author.

Needham, R. (1977). Casework intervention with a homosexual adolescent. *Social Casework, 58*(7), 387-394.

Newman, B. M. and Newman, P. R. (1987). *Development through life: A psychosocial approach,* fourth edition. Belmont, CA: Dorsey Press.

Newman, B. S. (1989). Including curriculum content on lesbian and gay issues. *Journal of Social Work Education, 25*(3), 202-211.

Nurius, P. and Hudson, W. (1988). Sexual activity and preference: Six quantifiable dimensions. *The Journal of Sex Research, 24,* 30-46.

Parr, R. G. and Jones, L. E. (1996). Point/counterpoint: Should CSWE allow social work programs in religious institutions an exemption from the accreditation nondiscrimination standard related to sexual orientation? *Journal of Social Work Education, 32*(3), 297-313.

Patterson, C. J. (1994). Lesbian and gay couples considering parenthood: An agenda for research, service and advocacy. In L. A. Kurdek (Ed.), *Social services for gay and lesbian couples,* (pp. 33-56). Binghamton, NY: Harrington Park Press.

Peplau, L. A. and Amaro, H. (1982). Understanding lesbian relationships. In W. Paul, J. D. Weinrich, J. C. Gonsiorek, and M. E. Hotvedt (Eds.), *Homosexuality: Social, psychological and biological issues* (pp. 233-248). Beverly Hills, CA: Sage Press.

Peterson, K. J. (Ed.). (1996). Health care for lesbians and gay men: Confronting homophobia and heterosexism. *Journal of Gay and Lesbian Social Services, 5*(1).

Pharr, S. (1988). *Homophobia: A weapon of sexism.* Little Rock, AK: Chardon Press.

Ponse, B. (1980). Finding self in the lesbian community. In M. Kirkpatrick (Ed.), *Women's sexual development* (pp. 181-200). New York: Plenum.

Potter, S. J. and Darty, T. E. (1981). Social work and the invisible minority: An exploration of lesbianism. *Social Work, 26*(3), 187-192.

Quam, J. (Ed.). (1997). *Social services for older gay men and lesbians.* Binghamton, NY: The Haworth Press.

Rabin, J., Keefe, K., and Burton, M. (1986). Enhancing services for sexual minority clients: A community mental health approach. *Social Work, 31*(4), 294-298.

Reiter, L. (1989). Sexual orientation, sexual identity, and the question of choice. *Clinical Social Work Journal, 17*(2), 138-150.

Reiter, L. (1991). Developmental origins of antihomosexual prejudice in heterosexual men and women. *Clinical Social Work Journal, 19*(2), 163-175.

Renzetti, C. M., and Miley, C. H. (Eds.). (1996). Violence in gay and lesbian domestic partnerships. [Special Issue]. *Journal of Gay and Lesbian Social Services, 4*(1).

Ricketts, W. and Achtenberg, R. (1990). Adoption and foster parenting for lesbians and gay men: Creating new traditions in family. *Marriage and Family Review, 14*(3/4), 83-118.

Rochlin, M. (1985). Sexual orientation of the therapist and therapeutic effectiveness with gay clients. In J. C. Gonsiorek (Ed.), *A guide to psychotherapy with gay and lesbian clients* (pp. 21-30). Binghamton, NY: Harrington Park Press.

Rogers, P. (1993 February 15). How many gays are there? *Newsweek,* p. 46.

Saghir, M. T., Robbins, E., and Walbian, B. (1973). *Male and female homosexuality: A comprehensive study.* Baltimore: Williams and Wilkins.

Salholz, E., Glick, D., Beachy, L., Monserrate, C., King, P., Gordon, J., and Barrett, T. (1993 June 21). The power and the pride: Lesbians, coming out strong. *Newsweek,* p. 54-60.

Sang, B. E. (1993). Existential issues of midlife lesbians. In L. D. Garnets and D. G. Kimmel (Eds.), *Psychological perspectives on lesbian and gay male experiences* (pp. 500-516). New York: Columbia University Press.

Savin-Williams, R. C. (1989). Gay and lesbian adolescents. *Marriage and Family Review, 14*(3-4), 197-216.

Schmalz, J. (1993a February 4). From midshipman to gay advocate. *The New York Times,* p. C1.

Schmalz, J. (1993b March 7). For gay people, a time of triumph and fear. *The New York Times*, p. L37.

Schmalz, J. (1993c May 7). In Hawaii, step toward legalized gay marriage. *The New York Times*, p. A14.

Schmitt, E. (1993a January 13). Clinton aides study indirect end to military ban on homosexuals. *The New York Times*, p. A1.

Schmitt, E. (1993b January 23). Joint chiefs fighting Clinton's plan to allow homosexuals in military. *The New York Times*, p. A1.

Schmitt, E. (1993c May 13). Family is unified in gay-ban debate. *The New York Times*, p. A1.

Schneider, M. (1988). *Often invisible: Counselling gay and lesbian youth.* Toronto: Toronto Central Youth Services.

Schneider, M. (1989). Sappho was a right-on adolescent. In G. Herdt (Ed.), *Gay and lesbian youth,* (pp. 111-130). Binghamton, NY: The Haworth Press.

Schneider, M. and Tremble, B. (1985). Gay or straight? Working with the confused adolescent. *Journal of Homosexuality, 4*(1/2), 71-82.

Schoenberg, R., Goldberg, R and Shore, D. (Eds.). (1985). *With compassion towards some: Homosexuality and social work in America.* New York: Harrington Park Press.

Scott, W. and Shernoff, M. (Eds.). (1988). *The source book on lesbian and gay health care.* Washington, DC: National Lesbian/Gay Health Foundation.

Shernoff, M. (1984). Family therapy for lesbian and gay clients. *Social Work, 29*(4), 393-396.

Shernoff, M. (1991). Eight years of working with people with HIV: Impact upon a therapist. In C. Silverstein (Ed.), *Gays, lesbians, and their therapists* (pp.227-239). New York: W.W. Norton and Co.

Shernoff, M. (1995). Male couples and their relationship styles. *Journal of Gay and Lesbian Social Services, 2*(2), 43-57.

Shernoff, M. (1996a). The last journey. *Family Therapy Networker, 3,* 35-41.

Shernoff, M. (Ed.). (1996b). *Human services for gay people: Clinical and community practice.* Binghamton, NY: The Haworth Press.

Shernoff, M. (1996c). Gay men choosing to be fathers. In M. Shernoff (Ed.), *Human services for gay people: Clinical and community pratice* (pp. 41-54). Binghamton, NY: Harrington Park Press.

Slater, S. (1995). *The lesbian family life cycle.* New York: The Free Press.

Sophie, J. (1985/1986). A critical examination of stage theories of lesbian identity development. *Journal of Homosexuality, 12*(3/4), 39-51.

Strommen, E. F. (1989). "You're a what?" Family member reactions to the disclosure of homosexuality. *Journal of Homosexuality, 18*(1/2), 37-58.

Sullivan, G. (Ed.). (1995). Gays and lesbians in Asia and the Pacific: Social and human services. [Special Issue]. *Journal of Gay and Lesbian Social Services, 2*(2).

Sullivan, T., and Schneider, M. (1987). Development and identity issues in adolescent homosexuality. *Child and Adolescent Social Work, 4*(1), 13-24.

Tafoya, T. (1992). Native gay and lesbian issues: The two-spirited. In B. Berzon, (Ed.), *Positively gay* (pp. 253-262). Berkeley, CA: Celestial Arts.

Teaching about gays and tolerance (1992 September 27). *The New York Times,* p. E16.

Tievsky, D. L. (1988). Homosexual clients and homophobic social workers. *Journal of Independent Social Work, 2*(3), 51-62.

Troiden, R. R. (1979). Becoming homosexual: A model of gay identity acquisition. *Psychiatry, 42,* 362-373.

Troiden, R. R. (1988). *Gay and lesbian identity: A sociological analysis.* Dix Hills, NY: General Hall, Inc.

Troiden, R. R. (1989). The formation of homosexual identities. In G. Herdt (Ed.), *Gay and lesbian youth* (pp. 43-74). Binghamton, NY: Harrington Park Press.

Tully, C. (Ed.). (1996). *Lesbian social services: Research issues.* Binghamton, NY: Harrington Park Press.

Tully, C. and Albro, J. C. (1979). Homosexuality: A social worker's imbroglio. *Journal of Sociology and Social Welfare, 6*(2), 154-167.

Vaughan, M. (1996 September 3). Dad's out and baby goes too. *The Glasgow Herald,* p. 11.

Wicks, L. K. (1978). Transsexualism: A social work approach. *Health and Social Work, 2*(1), 179-193.

Williams, L. (1993 June 28). Blacks reject gay rights fight as equal to theirs. *The New York Times.* p. A1.

Williams, W. (1986). *The spirit and the flesh: Sexual diversity in American Indian culture.* Boston: Beacon Press.

Williams, W. (1993). Persistence and change in the Berdache tradition among contemporary Lakota Indians. In L. D. Garnets and D. G. Kimmel (Eds.), *Psychological perspectives on lesbian and gay male experiences* (pp. 339-347). New York: Columbia University Press.

Wisniewski, J. J. and Toomey, B. G. (1987). Are social workers homophobic? *Social Work, 32*(5), 454-455.

Woodman, N. J. (Ed.). (1992). *Lesbian and gay lifestyles: A guide for counseling and education.* New York: Irvington.

Woodman, N., Tully, C. T., and Barranti, C. C. (1996). Research in lesbian communities: Ethical dilemmas. In C. Tully (Ed.), *Lesbian social services: Research issues* (pp. 57-66). Binghamton, NY: The Haworth Press.

Wyers, N. (1987). Homosexuality in the family: Lesbian and gay spouses. *Social Work, 32*(2), 143-149.

Zirin, J. D. (1996 September 3). Vows that could alter marriage. *The London Times,* p. 37.

Chapter 2

Values and Ethics in Social Work Practice with Lesbian and Gay Persons

Peg McCartt Hess
Howard J. Hess

The codified values and ethics of the profession reflect the heart and conscience of social work practice. In this chapter, we explore the profession's values and ethical principles as they relate to social work practice with lesbian and gay clients. In order to clearly focus our discussion on the profession's value and ethical commitments, this chapter is organized around six core values and related ethical principles as outlined in the current National Association of Social Workers (NASW) *Code of Ethics* (1996). Within each section, the discussion highlights ways in which social workers should incorporate the stated values and ethical principles in practice with gay men and lesbians and some of the obstacles that they may face in doing so. The chapter concludes with an identification of several frameworks useful in resolving ethical dilemmas.

Several recently revised professional documents identify the profession's core values and the expression and application of those values in practice. These include specific standards related to nondiscrimination against, social and economic justice for, and preparation for competent professional practice with a range of populations, including lesbians and gay men. The NASW *Code of Ethics,* revised and adopted by the Delegate Assembly of August 1996, states that social workers should ". . . obtain education about and seek to understand the nature of social diversity and oppression with respect to race, ethnicity, national origin, color, sex, sexual orientation, age, marital status, political belief, religion and mental or physical disability" (1.05(c)) and "act to prevent and eliminate domination, exploitation, and discrimination against any person, group, or class on the basis of . . . sexual orientation . . . or any other preference, personal characteristic, or status" (6.04(d)). The Council on Social Work Education (CSWE, 1992) *Curriculum Policy Statement,* revised and adopted by the CSWE Board in 1992, states that in both baccalaureate and master's programs, "The curriculum must provide content about people of color, women, and gay and lesbian persons" (pp. 101, 140). The recently revised CSWE *Evaluative Standards,* adopted by the board in 1994, states, "The program must be conducted without discrimination on the basis of . . . sexual orientation" (CSWE, 1994, pp. 84, 122).

Thus, the profession's commitment to prepare practitioners who demonstrate respect for the inherent dignity and worth of all persons and actively pursue social justice and social change on behalf of vulnerable and oppressed individuals and groups explicitly includes persons of differing sexual orientations. The realization of this commitment in social work education and practice, however, continues to challenge the profession as it attempts to move beyond the dictates and constraints of our homophobic and heterocentric social culture. In the following sections, these values and the related ethical principles are applied to practice with lesbian and gay persons.

THE PROFESSION'S CORE VALUES AND ETHICAL PRINCIPLES: APPLICATION IN PRACTICE WITH LESBIAN AND GAY CLIENTS

Consistent with the profession's historic and contemporary commitment to serving populations that are vulnerable and oppressed, the preamble of the NASW *Code of Ethics* (1996) states,

> The primary mission of the social work profession is to enhance human well-being and help meet basic human needs of all people, with particular attention to the needs and empowerment of people who are vulnerable, oppressed, and living in poverty. An historic and defining feature of social work is the profession's focus on individual well-being in a social context and the well-being of society. Fundamental to social work is

attention to the environmental forces that create, contribute to, and address problems in living.

. . . The mission of the social work profession is rooted in a set of core values. These core values, embraced by social workers throughout the profession's history, are the foundation of social work's unique purpose and perspective:

- Service
- Social justice
- Dignity and worth of the person
- Importance of human relationships
- Integrity
- Competence

The constellation of these core values reflects what is unique to the social work profession. Core values, and the principles which flow from them, must be balanced within the context and complexity of the human experience.

VALUE: *Service*
Ethical Principle: *Social workers' primary goal is to help people in need and to address social problems.*

Simply stated, the core value of service and the related goal of helping are the *sina quo non* of the social work profession. This simplicity, however, can be misleading. The determinations concerning whom, how, where, and in what ways one serves and what in fact is experienced by others as helpful are often complex and challenging to make. As introduced in the first chapter in this volume and discussed throughout, a client's sexual orientation may or may not be known to the practitioner and in some instances may be a matter of confusion and/or shame to the client. Therefore, in order to serve and be helpful, social work practitioners must be able to connect with persons who are lesbian and gay. Establishing such connections requires agency and practitioner messages that convey authentic inclusivity, acceptance, and affirmation; recognition of the varying role of sexual orientation in an individual client's service needs and of the range of appropriate interventive options; and understanding of the relationship between the experiences of individual lesbians and gay men and the homophobic heterocentric culture in which they live.

First, in aspiring to serve and help individual lesbian and gay persons, their family members and friends, and the lesbian and gay community, social work practitioners and agencies that employ them must critically examine the degree to which their services are truly accessible. Enacting the professional value of service requires an organizational and individual professional commitment to intentional inclusivity in the development of policies, programs, and practices that are "user friendly" to lesbian and gay clients and couples, families headed by gay and lesbian parents, and families with gay and lesbian family members. Agency brochures, forms, and other written materials should portray images of gay and lesbian staff and clientele. Particular attention must be given to the use of nonheterocentric language in telephone and in-person transactions between staff and potential clients. For example, changing the question "Are you married?" to "Do you have a partner?" conveys openness and the capacity to help lesbian and gay clients as individuals and as couples. In a discussion of the promotion of organizational environments that are "user friendly" to all family forms, Hess and Jackson (1995) state,

> . . . the questions that families are asked directly and on intake forms either encourage clients to acknowledge openly their families' unique membership and set of relationships, roles, and needs or convey the assumption that client families must be traditionally constituted. Questions should anticipate that children may be biological, step-, adopted, or foster children or members of the extended family (nieces or nephews) and that they may have one caregiver (a single mother or father, a grandmother, an aunt, or a godparent), two caregivers, (such as a mother and a father, a mother and a mother, a father and a father, a mother and an aunt, or a grandmother and a grandfather), or two or more parents in separate household who share joint custody. Social workers must be mindful that simple questions about family membership can be posed in ways that shame or alienate the client or encourage deception. (pp. 134-135)

Helping persons who are lesbian and gay also requires skill in assessing with the client whether sexual orientation is in the foreground or background of her or his concern and service need. An assumption that sexual orientation would be in the foreground conveys the practitioner's misconception that being lesbian or gay is a "problem." On the other hand, a practitioner's assumption that sexual orientation would be irrelevant conveys a lack of understanding of the many ways in which the client's life experience is affected by the homophobic reactions of family members, friends, employers, and her or his own internalized homophobia. The discussions throughout this volume provide ample illustration of these and of the range of interventive options that may prove helpful.

Serving persons who are lesbian and gay also requires that organizations and practitioners identify and address social problems that affect them individually and collectively. These include discrimination in employment, in health and other benefits, in educational settings, and in family courts, as well as violence perpetrated against gay and lesbian persons. Addressing such problems requires social workers to advocate with and on behalf of lesbian and gay clients, be vigilant against institutional discrimination against gay and lesbian clients, and be visible in joining with the lesbian and gay communities to address community and social problems.

The following vignette illustrates the relevance of these dimensions. A young couple, Ray and Jolene, sought help from a family service agency. Initially they identified concerns with the behavior of their four-year-old daughter Roxanne, who was attending day care. Day care staff reported that she was hitting other children, was unable to relax during nap time, and had frequent temper tantrums. Ray and Jolene were concerned that the center might refuse continued service, affecting their ability to retain their employment. The social worker engaged with Jolene and Ray to assess Roxanne's behaviors, the tensions with the marital relationship, and both parents' satisfaction with their lives. Ray was struggling with a worsening depression that he attributed to a growing distance between himself and Jolene, a distance he couldn't explain. Several times Jolene mentioned being unable to be herself in the relationship and alluded to a secret that she couldn't share. Through a skillful series of individual and joint discussions, the social worker was able to help Jolene acknowledge the reality of her lesbian sexual orientation and share this with Ray. With the secret out, the social worker, Jolene, and Ray began to identify and work together on the many decisions that each faced individually and as parents. In reflecting upon their initial call to this particular family service agency, Jolene noted having seen a brochure in Roxanne's pediatrician's office describing the agency's service, including a group on parenting issues for lesbian and gay parents. Once connected to the agency, Jolene had experienced the social worker as open in her ongoing assessment of the range of possible sources of Jolene's expressed ability to "be herself" in her relationship with Ray.

VALUE: *Social Justice*
Ethical Principle: *Social workers challenge social injustice.*

Historically and currently, the social work profession is strongly identified with the value of social justice. Challenging injustice and pursuing social change are integral to each professional social worker's job description. As described in Chapter 1 and throughout this volume, homophobia and heterocentrism are powerful and insidious forces that have resulted in discrimination and inequality for gay and lesbian persons in many aspects of their lives.

Social workers have an ethical responsibility to be informed about the degree to which gay and lesbian persons in their communities are ensured equality of opportunity and access to needed information, services, resources, and meaningful participation in decision making. Social workers must use their professional knowledge, skills, and influence to enhance equal opportunity and access. As asserted by Hartman, "On the national level, we must press NASW to more actively take on the issue of gay rights and to make the weight of our profession felt by those who would reverse the movement toward acceptance and equity for gay men and lesbians" (1993, p. 360).

Informing oneself about one's own organization's policies, programs, and practices is a responsible beginning point. What are lesbian and gay clients' experiences in the school, community mental health clinic, family service agency, residential treatment facility, hospital, shelter, or other setting in which you are employed or are placed as a social work intern? In your community, what are the experiences of people who are lesbian and gay when they seek to access health benefits for themselves and/or their families, run for president of the local high school student council or of the school's PTA, become licensed as a foster parent, volunteer as a Big Brother or a Big Sister, adopt a child, join a health club, attend parenting classes, or apply for a mortgage?

In practice with lesbian and gay clients it is important to recognize the close relationship between case and cause. Given the extent to which oppression is ever present in the lives of persons who are gay and lesbian, it is often essential to include advocacy as a service component. The following example illustrates this point. A child care agency in a metropolitan community was concerned about the length of time spent by "hard to place" infants and young children in foster care and institutional settings. Identified as hard to place because of special medical, physical, and emotional needs, the children typically required extensive parental involvement in daily care and parental involvement with a range of professionals. In response to the agency's outreach to potential adoptive parents, a number of single gay men and lesbians and gay and lesbian couples applied. Some applicants were parents; others, in adopting a child, would become a parent for the first time. Following extensive assessment of the applicant pool, the agency selected several persons who were gay and lesbian for preadoptive placement preparation and planning. Upon challenges from other applicants in the pool regarding their selection, the agency stated the position that it would not discriminate against applicants on the basis of sexual orientation. A number of individuals and groups subsequently approached agency administrators and staff, portraying the lesbian and gay applicants as wishing to "convert" children to their sexual orientation and accusing the agency of subjecting children to a "deviant" lifestyle. Recognizing that both the well-being of the applicants and of the children were at stake, agency administrators, supervisors, and staff in the program engaged in both education and advocacy. For example, staff initiated meetings with members of the agency's board, social workers in key positions in the community, and other influential community professionals to provide information, respond to concerns, and secure support. Several national organizations were contacted by agency staff in order to identify educational resources and individuals available for consultation. The PBS documentary "We Are Family" (Sands, 1986), which depicts gay and lesbian parents and their biological, foster, and adoptive children, was provided to community agencies and professional groups. While recognizing some risk to community support of the agency, the staff concluded that the issue of social justice must be confronted. The program remained intact and efforts to prevent the placements of children with lesbian and gay parents were thwarted.

VALUE: *Dignity and Worth of the Person*
Ethical Principle: *Social workers respect the inherent dignity and worth of the person.*

Respect for the dignity and worth of all people is perhaps the most basic of social work values. However, its application in practice with lesbian and gay persons requires a profound commitment to self-determination and strong skills in facilitating the enhancement of self-esteem in others. As articulated in the NASW *Code of Ethics,* "Social workers respect and promote the right of clients to self-determination and assist clients in their efforts to identify and clarify their goals" (p. 12).

In promoting the self-determination of their lesbian and gay clients, some social workers may confront a sense of dissonance as they weigh their professional knowledge, their personal beliefs, their feelings for their clients, and professional standards. Valuing the dignity and worth of each person is a matter of thinking, feeling, and acting. Although our respect for the inherent dignity and worth of persons who are lesbian, gay, bisexual, and transgendered is primarily demonstrated through our professional behaviors, our capacity to behave respectfully is inevitably shaped by our personal experiences and values, professional knowledge and training, openness to feedback from others, and personal and professional commitment to a disciplined use of self.

Internalized homophobia and heterocentrism often undermine a gay and lesbian clients' own sense of value and self-worth. In some instances, a client's confusion about her or his sexual orientation potentially undermines self-determination and clarity about life goals. In such instances, the practitioner's expression of respect for the client's struggle, potential, and worth must be unwavering. The following vignette demonstrates a social worker's skill in communicating his valuing of a young gay client.

Joshua began meeting with a social worker in his high school at the age of fifteen. He was experiencing depression, insomnia, and difficulties in completing his schoolwork. After finding male pornographic magazines on the kitchen table, Joshua's sister asked Joshua is they were his. In the course of their conversation, Joshua acknowledged his attraction to other boys. His sister urged him to "talk with someone." After several further conversations with his sister, Joshua "stopped by" to talk with the social worker who had presented in several of his health classes about different problems that teenagers confront, including suicidal thoughts and confusion about sexual orientation. The social worker began meeting with Joshua and learned that Joshua had always felt different. The youngest in his family, he loved dancing and acting and had participated in a number of stage productions in school and summer camp. His father had discouraged these activities and had found reasons to avoid attending most of the events in which Joshua performed. He described having kissed several girls and having felt nothing. He told the social worker he believed he might be gay, but had discussed his feelings with no one. He was deeply distressed about his belief that his father was disappointed in him. He was experiencing increased attractions to men and a recurring sense of panic in his isolation from family and friends. The social worker concluded that Joshua was confused and sad about accepting himself as a gay man. He helped Joshua initiate a discussion with his mother about his belief that he might be gay. Though initially frightened by this disclosure, his mother was reassured that Joshua had confided in her. The social worker actively engaged in helping Joshua assess and recognize his inherent worth and value, clarifying and then challenging the negative self-statements that characterized Joshua's conversations with him. The social worker also facilitated Joshua's participation in a group of gay, lesbian, and bisexual youth in the community. Through an intricate process involving conversations with the social worker, his mother and sister, and other gay, lesbian, and bisexual youth, Joshua was able to begin to express hopefulness about his life and his worth. He began to construct a self-concept as a bright, talented, and sensitive young man. As he became clearer about his sexual orientation and his identity, he began to come out to his friends and, with the support of his mother and his sister, to his father. His relationships and academic work began to stabilize. He maintained his connection to the social worker as he began to explore the transition from high school and family to college.

VALUE: *Importance of Human Relationships*
Ethical Principle: *Social workers recognize the central importance of human relationships.*

Social workers understand that human development, change, and opportunity occur within the context of nurturing, accepting, and supportive relationships. Perhaps the greatest cost of homophobia occurs in relationships. Therefore, a central focus of practice with persons who are lesbian and gay is on relationships–bringing honesty into relationships, reducing tensions in relationships, redefining or ending relationships, and developing new relationships.

In practicing with lesbian and gay persons, it is important to recognize the vital importance of supportive social networks. Reflective of the social isolation faced by many lesbians and gay men, close interpersonal ties are often limited or constrained. As illustrated by the situations described previously, intimate relationships with parents, siblings, children, and friends may become compromised and incomplete. Many lesbian and gay clients need assistance in healing current relationships and/or in developing new relationships in order to decrease their sense of isolation, achieve their goals, and enhance their well-being. The following vignette demonstrates the potency of group intervention in working with gay men who are HIV positive.

A community-based HIV/AIDS service organization recognized the social isolation experienced by many gay men newly diagnosed with HIV infection. Fearful of disclosure to families, co-workers, and sometimes even close friends, this population of clients grew increasingly fearful and depressed. In addition to case management, emergency financial aid, and buddy services, the agency initiated several support groups for recently diagnosed HIV-positive men. The purpose of the groups was defined as mutual aid. Group membership was voluntary and expected to change depending on members' needs. Meeting on a weekly basis, one of the groups consisted of approximately twenty-two members, including two HIV-negative partners. Cofacilitated by one of the authors as a volunteer, a simple format was used in which each member briefly checked in and an agenda was developed from those items. Occasionally, lecturers were invited into the group and social events were scheduled. However, the simple process of sharing openly in a safe place where confidentiality was assured set in motion a powerful process of mutual support and caring. Members reported their struggles with health issues, unresponsive professional caregivers, struggles with families and partners, and fears about death. As a result, members achieved a level of intimacy with one another unlike that found in most areas of their lives. Many group members described the group as their substitute family. Over time, group members developed familylike practices such as having a Thanksgiving buffet on Thanksgiving eve and dinner together on Christmas Day. Many group members had been estranged from their immediate and extended families for long periods of time. Most members identified this estrangement as more related to being gay than to being HIV positive.

Group members often planned other social activities, including traveling to see the AIDS Quilt and developing several fundraising events. As the group members developed friendships based on honest expressions of their identities, fears, and needs, members reported an increase in positive self-esteem and an overall sense of empowerment. As some group members became ill and subsequently died, they were supported through these experiences by other members of the group. Many reported that their capacity to confront illness, pain, and possible death was greatly enhanced by helping others and knowing that others were committed to helping them. Group members came to trust that they were not alone.

VALUE: *Integrity*
Ethical Principle: *Social workers behave in a trustworthy manner.*

The NASW *Code of Ethics* rightfully holds that social workers should aspire to be trustworthy in all professional activities. When working with lesbians and gay men, integrity is particularly crucial to effective practice. Given the extent to which matters of sexual orientation have been cloaked in secrecy, it is often unrealistic to expect that openness and clarity will be present with our clients, our colleagues, or even within ourselves. The pervasive presence of homophobia in our society has tended to discourage these qualities. Consequently, in a purposeful way, professional social workers must engage in a process of self-examination and change that in turn will contribute to the creation of more trustworthy professional relationships with clients and trustworthy programs and organizations for gay and lesbian clients.

The ongoing process of developing self-awareness is central to integrity in practice with persons who are lesbian and gay. In spite of the general professional social work awareness that discrimination on the basis of sexual orientation is unacceptable, basic attitudes about persons who are lesbian and gay continue to be strongly influenced by homophobia. It is reasonable to expect that just as all persons reared in our culture have internalized some elements of racism, homophobia has been internalized as well. This is often as true for lesbian and gay persons as for those who are heterosexual. Consequently, it is imperative that professional social workers challenge their own attitudes and beliefs about sexual orientation through a process of systematic self-exploration. Social workers need to be comfortable with both the feminine and masculine aspects of themselves and be capable of empathy with clients whose emotional lives and sexual orientation are similar to or different from their own. For all social workers, it is important to explore one's own sexual orientation fully in order not to displace upon clients issues that grow out of one's own concerns and life experiences. Whatever one's own sexual orientation, it is important to be able to accept and tolerate the variety of choices that may be made by lesbian and gay clients about self-disclosure to family, friends, co-workers, and others.

Issues of practitioner self-disclosure regarding sexual orientation have both practice and ethical dimensions. For practitioners who are themselves lesbian or gay, practice with gay and lesbian clients may present particular challenges as discussed in several of the chapters in this collection. Particularly in small communities, the ethical directives concerning dual or multiple relationships with clients or former clients and concerning clients' rights to privacy require attention and care.

Respect for the confidential nature of practice with persons who are lesbian and gay is essential to the definition of trustworthiness. While all clients are rightfully concerned about privacy and confidentiality, clients who are gay and lesbian are likely to be acutely sensitive to the nature of information shared among agency co-workers and maintained in agency records and practitioners' personal notes. Davidson and Davidson (1996) thoughtfully describe the vulnerability of clients in a "culture of information processing" (p. 215). Confidential information regarding clients' sexual orientation must be carefully protected. Social workers should question under what circumstances information concerning the sexual orientation of clients should be recorded and maintained as a part of agency records, particularly when information is to be passed on to managed care companies. Inadvertently "outing" a client or client's family member is tantamount to betrayal and an egregious breach of professional ethics.

VALUE: *Competence*
Ethical Principle: *Social workers practice within their areas of competence and develop and enhance their professional expertise.*

It is the expectation of the National Association of Social Workers that professionals should limit their practice to those areas in which they have established a necessary degree of competence. However, such a principle should not provide an easy rationale for refusing to work with lesbians and gay men. Rather, we agree with the standard established by the Council on Social Work Education in 1992 that preparation for social work practice fundamentally must include practice with lesbians and gay men. Competence must be established through mastery of a knowledge base about practice with lesbians and gay men, having an exposure to gay and lesbian clients during internship experiences, and investing in exploration of one's own homophobia, stereotypes, and personal beliefs and biases.

As a component of professional education, content regarding the historic and current life experiences of gays and lesbians is essential. It is beyond the scope of this chapter to delineate the knowledge requisite to achieve competent practice with persons who are gay and lesbian, but key components include the following:

- Individual human development, including the androgynous, dual gender characteristics of all persons
- The developmental milestones for lesbian and gay persons, such as the coming-out experience, and the essential characteristics of lesbian and gay identity development as evidenced through the life stories now available in print (Alyson, 1991; Due, 1995; Heron, 1994; Kay, Estepa, and Desetta, 1996; Miranda, 1996; Monette, 1992).
- The extensive literature regarding the source of sexual orientation, including genetics (See LeVey, 1991)
- The typical concerns of lesbian and gay couples (See McVinney and Barranti's chapters in this collection) and developmental cycles of lesbian and gay families
- The struggle for human rights by the lesbian and gay communities (See Vaid, 1995).
- The study of and opportunity to apply assessment and intervention strategies for practice with lesbian and gay clients and their families (See Mallon, Chapter 7 in this collection)
- The study of and opportunity to apply knowledge about exemplary programs for members of the lesbian and gay communities, such as programs for lesbian and gay youth (Mallon, in press)

A strength of social work education is the opportunity to test theory in supervised practice. These authors propose that all students should have the opportunity to practice with lesbian and gay clients. It is anticipated that issues will arise related to students' homophobia, heterocentrism, and self-disclosure. Some students will struggle in practice and gain extensively from such a learning opportunity. In some instances, this opportunity will result in a better understanding of a student's appropriateness for the profession. For example, a first-year student in a large social work MSW program in the western part of the United States recently conferred with one of the authors about his unwillingness to provide counseling to a gay couple as a part of his field practicum. He had refused to do so based upon his religious beliefs, which defined any gay sexual behavior as sinful. After lengthy discussions, this student had been asked to leave the school because it was decided that he was inappropriate for the profession of social work. The author's response was that the student's refusal to practice in any way with lesbian and gay clients was deeply inconsistent with the value base of the profession. It is recognized that students will grow and develop in the learning process; however, a basic unwillingness to work fully with clients of both genders, multiple races and ethnicities, and differing sexual orientations is a necessary condition for entry into the profession.

IDENTIFYING, ANALYZING, AND RESOLVING ETHICALLY CHALLENGING PRACTICE PROBLEMS AND DILEMMAS

Although in most situations the core values and related ethical principles identified in the profession's code of ethics are sufficient to shape and direct practice decisions, in some situations ethical dilemmas or conflict emerge. The professional literature provides numerous discussions of these, and in many agencies and settings ethics committees have been established to provide guidance to professionals confronting such dilemmas. Several resources include guidelines for ethical decision making and are highly recommended. These include *Social Work Values and Ethics* (Reamer, 1995); *Ethical Decisions for Social Work Practice* (Lowenberg and Dolgoff, 1996); and *Ethical Dilemmas in Social Work Practice* (Rhodes, 1986).

CONCLUSION

Social work practice with persons who are gay and lesbian must be infused with the core set of professional values and shaped by ethical principles. Given social work's commitment to serve oppressed populations, this area of practice is central for the profession. A set of core values and ethical principles has been explicated in this essay and provides one approach to developing a practice approach that is sensitive to issues of sexual orientation.

REFERENCES

Alyson, S. (Ed.). (1991). *Young, gay and proud.* Boston: Alyson Publications.

Council on Social Work Education. (1992). *Curriculum policy statement for master's degree programs in social work education.* Alexandria, VA: Council on Social Work Education (CSWE).

Council on Social Work Education Commission on Accreditation. (1994). *Handbook of accreditation standards and procedures*, fourth edition. Alexandria, VA: CSWE.

Davidson, J. R. and Davidson, T. (1996). Confidentiality and managed care: Ethical and legal concerns. *Health and Social Work, 21,* 208-215.

Due, L. (1995). *Joining the tribe: Growing up gay and lesbian in the 90's.* New York: Anchor Books.

Hartman, A. (1993). Out of the closet: Revolution and backlash. *Social Work, 38*(3), 245-246,360.

Heron, A. (Ed.). (1994). *Two teenagers in 20.* Boston: Alyson Publications.

Hess, P. M. and Jackson, H. (1995). Practice with and on behalf of families. In C. Meyer and M. Mattaini (Eds.), *The foundations of social work practice* (126-155). Washington, DC: National Association of Social Workers.

Kay, P., Estepa, A., and Desetta, A. (Eds.). (1996). *Out with it: Gay and straight teens write about homosexuality.* New York: Youth Communications.

LeVey, S. (1991 August 31). A difference in hypothalmic structure between heterosexual and homosexual men. *Science, 253* (5023), pp. 1034-1037.

Lowenberg, F.M. and Dolgoff, R. (1996). *Ethical decisions for social work practice*, fourth edition. Itasca, IL: F.E. Peacock.

Mallon, G. P. (in press). Entering into a collaborative search for meaning with gay and lesbian youths in out-of-home care: An empowerment-based model for training child welfare professionals. *Child and Adolescent Social Work Journal.*

Miranda, D. (1996). I hated myself. In P. Kay, A. Estepa, and A. Desetta (Eds.), *Out with it: Gay and straight teens write about homosexuality* (pp. 34-39). New York: Youth Communications.

Monette, P. (1992). *Becoming a man: Half a life story.* New York: Harcourt Brace Jovanovich.

National Association of Social Workers. (1996) *Code of ethics.* Washington, DC: NASW Press.

Reamer, F. (1995). *Social work values and ethics.* New York: Columbia University Press.

Rhodes, M. (1986). *Ethical dilemmas in social work practice.* Boston: Routledge and Kegan Paul.

Sands, A. (Producer). (1986). *We are family.* Boston: WGBH.

Vaid, U. (1995). *Virtual equality: The mainstreaming of gay and lesbian liberation.* New York: Anchor books.

Chapter 3

Negotiating Conflicts in Allegiances Among Lesbians and Gays of Color: Reconciling Divided Selves and Communities

Karina L. Walters

I used to wonder why I have so often felt preoccupied with issues of boundary and identity. Why am I still startled when someone asks, yet again . . . are you a woman first or a person of color/Asian American first? . . . [or] if this is a lesbian group, why do you keep talking about race? We are all women here . . . How does one negotiate a multiple-situated identity if race, gender, and sexual orientation are taken for granted as so separate and boundaried? (Karen Maeda Allman, 1996, p. 277)

The successful development of healthy group and self identities among members of oppressed groups involves the ability to reconcile competing demands from the dominant society and the individual's ethnic, racial, or gay and lesbian community. Research (Helms, 1989; Phinney, 1990; Sue, 1992; Walters and Simoni, 1993) has demonstrated that positive gay and lesbian self and group identities as well as a positive racial or ethnic identity are integrally connected to psychological well-being. Despite the recognition that ethnic or gay identity is important in mental health functioning, little research has investigated the multiple oppressed statuses and the interactions

The author gratefully acknowledges Jane Simoni, PhD, for her editorial and conceptual contributions to this chapter.

of those statuses on psychosocial functioning among gays and lesbians of color (GALOCs). For GALOCs, the integration of a consolidated racial and gay or lesbian identity is even more complex, involving negotiations of conflicting allegiances to the gay and lesbian community and their community of color. Despite the importance of understanding the complex interactions among racism, sexism, and heterosexism that GALOCs must negotiate, the social work practice literature remains inadequate in providing any practice guidelines that incorporate these issues.

This chapter explores how racial and gay/lesbian identities moderate life stressors associated with a double or triple oppressed group status and the conflicts in allegiances that arise as a result of these life stressors. At the end of the chapter, implications for social work individual and community practice will be discussed from an ecological life-modeled perspective (Germain and Gitterman, 1996).

To simply cluster all GALOCs into a homogenous category is misleading. GALOCs come from very diverse backgrounds (e.g., American Indian, African American, Latino/a, and Asian American), and, as a result, there is greater diversity within groups than there is between groups (Sue, 1992). For the purposes of this work, the term GALOCs refer to those individuals who self-identify primarily monoracially (e.g., African American) and monosexually (e.g., as gay or lesbian). Although the issues facing bisexuals of color and multiracial gays and lesbians will be at times discussed, a further explication of specific issues facing multiracial bisexuals, multiracial gays and lesbians, and bisexuals of color are even more complex and deserve greater in-depth examination. For an excellent preliminary discussion of these issues see Allman (1996), Greene (1993), Kich (1996), and Root (1996).

In most mental health research, one of two dialectic frameworks frequently predominate: the universalist approach (etic) or a cultural-relativist approach (emic). The epistemological presentation of issues facing GALOCs is a fusion of these approaches. The focus of this chapter will be on identifying the universal process involved in negotiating conflicts in allegiances across racial groups and highlighting culture-specific manifestations of the universal process for specific racial groups. Although the thrust of this chapter is on identifying universal processes, it is important that practitioners utilize this perspective only as a guide, integrating universal processes with the GALOC's culture-specific experience. Identifying only universal processes neglects the specificity of the GALOC's sociohistorical-cultural experience.

PREVIOUS RESEARCH ON RACIAL IDENTITY, GAY/LESBIAN IDENTITY, AND GALOC IDENTITY

There is evidence that a parallel process of racial, ethnic, and sexual-orientation identity development exists for oppressed populations, involving movement from internalized negative attitudes about self and group to an integrated identity (Cross, 1978; Helms, 1990; Parham and Helms, 1985a, 1985b; Phinney, 1990). Previous research suggests that mental health outcomes such as depression and self-esteem are moderated by one's positive or negative group and self identity attitudes (Walters, 1995; Walters and Simoni, 1993). Although prior research has focused on how identity attitudes moderate various mental health outcomes, it is assumed here that a parallel process occurs whereby GALOC identity attitudes moderate the relationship between conflicts in allegiances and mental health outcomes (e.g., anxiety or depression).

Collapsing the different ethnic/racial identity stage models, a progression emerges that stands as a standard framework in which identity-attitude processes evolve (Atkinson, Morten, and Sue, 1983; Cross; 1978; Parham and Helms, 1985a, 1985b; Phinney, 1990; Sue, 1992; Walters, 1995). For example, the urban American Indian identity model (UAII) (Walters, 1995), like other racial identity models, consists of four stages (i.e., internalization, marginalization, externalization, actualization) that tap into a process of identity development from internalized oppression and self/group deprecation to a positive, integrated self and group identity (Walters, 1995). According to the UAII model, identity attitudes are formed in the context of the person (self identity), the person's group (group identity), the person's social environment (urban environment), and the historical relationship with the dominant society (dominant group environment and institutional responses).

Research on GALOCs and their concurrent identity development have been conducted on small samples of African Americans (Hendin, 1969; Icard, 1986; Johnson, 1982; Loiacano, 1989), Mexican Americans (Espin, 1987; Morales, 1989), and Asian Americans (Chan, 1989; Wooden, Kawaksaki, and Mayeda, 1983). Researchers (Walters, 1997) studying GALOC identity generally combine the racial and ethnic identity attitude models (i.e., Atkinson, Morten, and Sue, 1983; Cross, 1978; Helms, 1990; Parham and Helms, 1985a, 1985b; Phinney, 1990; Sue, 1992) with Cass's (1984) gay and lesbian identity model.

The GALOC identity research describes two orthogonal processes that occur simultaneously, one in terms of racial identity and the other in terms of the acquisition of a gay or lesbian self identity via the coming out process (Walters, 1997). The racial identity models focus on group identity and the corresponding attitudes that one has toward one's own group, whereas the "coming out" models focus on the awareness of self identity and coming to terms with the realization of being gay. For example, Morales (1989) proposed a five-state model of ethnic gay and lesbian identity that consists of (a) a denial of conflicts in allegiances, (b) coming out as bisexual versus gay/lesbian, (c) conflicts in allegiances, (d) establishing priorities in allegiances, and (e) integration of identities.

However, none of the GALOC identity models addresses ethnic gay or lesbian identity as it changes over time throughout adulthood (i.e., post-"coming out" as gay or lesbian) nor do they examine the psychological attitudes that GALOCs have toward gays and lesbians as a group (i.e., group identity attitudes [Walters, 1997]). The trend in identity research suggests that a multilevel, multidimensional approach must explore self and group identity attitudes across both gay/lesbian group membership as well as racial group membership. GALOC's identity must be understood within this multilevel context.

In this chapter, the GALOC identity matrix model expands upon the earlier racial and gay identity models and the model proposed by Walters (1997) for gay and lesbian American Indians (i.e., the GLAI model) and acts as a means to demonstrate the identity adaptation of GALOCS; second, the author presents a stress-coping paradigm and discusses its implications for practice. Both conceptual models are needed for effective practice with GALOCs.

APPLYING THE LIFE MODEL:
THE STRESS-COPING PROCESS REVISITED

Life-modeled practice is derived in part from Lazarus' (1980) stress-coping paradigm. This work expands on the traditional understanding of the stress-coping process, adding a moderating factor that strengthens positive coping responses for GALOCs.

Germain and Gitterman (1996) point out that external life stressors and their corresponding internal stress are manifestations of negative transactions between the person and the environment. Life stressors are externally generated (e.g., racism) and can become internalized (e.g., internalized racism). Additionally, life stressors can take the form of anticipated rejection by others or potential loss. The consequences of these life stressors can then be experienced as an internal stressor affecting emotional and psychological well-being (Germain and Gitterman, 1996). At times, stress can become immobilizing or become expressed as hopelessness, helplessness, powerlessness, anxiety, guilt, ambivalence, or despair (Germain and Gitterman, 1996).

A critical task that GALOCs face is to reconcile the conflicts in allegiances that arise as the result of being a member of two oppressed groups (i.e., gay men of color) or three oppressed groups (i.e., as women, lesbians, and persons of color) (Chan, 1989; Greene, 1994; Hendin, 1969; Icard, 1986; Johnson, 1982; Loiacano, 1989; Morales, 1989). GALOCs participate in disparate social worlds, which include their gay and lesbian community, their community of color, and the dominant culture (i.e., heterosexuals and white Americans [Walters, 1996]). To walk in multiple worlds requires the ability to traverse many social and cultural boundaries and multiple social roles and expectations and, as a result, involves encountering multiple levels of stressors. Thus, GALOCs experience discrimination within their own culture (i.e., heterosexism as a gay man or a lesbian); within the gay and lesbian community (racism as a racial minority); and within the dominant group (heterosexism and racism as both a gay male and as an ethnic person; or heterosexism and racism and sexism as an ethnic person, a woman, and a lesbian).

PARADIGM OF THE STRESS PROCESS

Dinges and Joos (1988) expanded upon a prior model of stress and coping to include antecedents of stressful life events in the conceptualization of client process (Dohrenwend and Dohrenwend, 1981). In their modified model, they identified environmental contexts and person factors as the antecedents of stressful life events, which lead to varying states of stress (Dinges and Joos, 1988). Positive, neutral, or negative wellness outcomes depend upon the interaction of internal factors (e.g., identity attitudes) with the state of stress. Additionally, the vulnerability hypothesis posits that associations between life events and adverse health/mental health changes are moderated by preexisting personal dispositions (e.g., identity attitudes) that function as buffers, making individuals psychologically and emotionally strong (Dinges and Joos, 1988). Dinges and Joos found this model to be the most effective for depicting stress, coping, and health/mental health relationships for Indian populations and expect that this model can be generalized to other oppressed populations.

This work incorporates a heuristic model that examines how GALOC identity attitudes moderate (i.e., have an interactive effect upon) the relation between life stressors (i.e., heterosexism, sexism, racism in creating conflicts in allegiances) and mental health outcomes for GALOCs. Morales (1989) reports that difficulties in integrating conflicts in allegiances may lead to heightened feelings of anxiety, tension, depression, isolation, anger, and problems in integrating aspects of self. Moreover, the potential rejection or perceived loss of support from one's own ethnic community compromises one's much needed social support, coping assistance, and survival skills. Identification of this process will assist social work practitioners in facilitating healthy GALOCs coping in response to the demands of their various communities

HETEROSEXISM, RACISM, AND SEXISM: CREATING CONFLICTS IN ALLEGIANCES

Similar to multiracial individuals, GALOCs challenge preconceived notions of group membership and assumptions associated with racial and sexual orientation status. For example, Root (1996) states that race is socially constructed in terms of the perspective of the power holder, generally forcing blended individuals (e.g., GA-LOCs) to artificially pick which "side" they belong to. Moreover, Root (1996) notes that:

> These experiences are not solely imposed by European-descended individuals; they are imposed from all sides in a manner that can choke the blended individual with a squeeze of oppression in the form of "authenticity tests," forced choices, or unwarranted assumptions about one's identity. (p. 20)

Although the functions and processes of both racism and heterosexism begin with those in power, the process can be internalized by oppressed groups and is manifested in the insistence on singular racial or sexual orientation loyalties (Root, 1996). For example, Audre Lorde (1984) writes,

> Differences between ourselves as black women are also being misnamed and used to separate us from one another. As a black lesbian feminist comfortable with the many different ingredients of my identity, and as a women committed to racial and sexual freedom from oppression, I find I am constantly being encouraged to pluck out some one aspect of myself and present this as a meaningful whole, eclipsing or denying the other parts of self. But this is a destructive and fragmenting way to live. (p. 63)

Thus, similar to multiracial individuals, GALOCs are constantly confronted with questions about their allegiances and forced to side with one group or the other. In essence, GALOCs deconstruct and challenge by their very presence the traditional assumptions of uni-lateral oppressed group membership.

Tests of Group Loyalty

Root (1996) points out that tests of loyalty and group member-ship legitimacy are always power struggles reflecting the internal-ization of colonized group thinking. Audre Lorde (1984) reminds us that as a tool of social control, oppressed groups are socialized to recognize only one aspect of their experience as salient for the survival of the group. Moreover, Lorde notes that we live in a society in which there is an institutionalized and socialized rejection of within-group differences. Our refusal to recognize our within-group differences and to investigate the distortions that arise from our misnaming these differences results in oppressive conditions for individuals with multiple situated identities (e.g., GALOCs [Lorde, 1984]).

THE ROOT OF CONFLICTS IN ALLEGIANCES: PRESSURES FOR UNITY VIA HOMOGENEITY

Lorde states that often members of oppressed groups identify by only one dimension of being oppressed and generalize that one dimension as being the only salient category of oppression for the entire group. As a result, many who experience one form of oppression as primary forget that members of "their" group may be experiencing multiple oppressed statuses and that they themselves might be oppressors to these individuals (Lorde, 1984). Thus, there is an intense pressure for homogeneity within groups that is confused with the need for group unity for survival purposes (i.e., for the fight against racism and genocide [Lorde, 1984]). As a result, group unity is confounded with group homogeneity. The result of this misnaming is the internalized divide-and-conquer mentality. A colonized mentality assumes that individuals who embrace their multiple identities and fight corresponding interlocking oppressions are dangerous to the group's unity and survival. Because of the continuous battle against genocide, the disavowal to recognize and name the within-group oppressions such as sexism and heterosexism become the status quo (Lorde, 1984), and, in fact, are sometimes mislabeled as "cultural" norms. This internalized, colonized oppression often becomes the criterion within communities of color by which gender roles and group survival can be authenticated and measured (Lorde, 1984). Thus, hostility and oppression against GALOCs is practiced not only by white society and white lesbians and gays, but by heterosexual communities of color as well.

Racism in the Gay and Lesbian Community

Historically, strong institutional ties (e.g., National Gay and Lesbian Task Force) and businesses (e.g., bars, social clubs) of gay and lesbian communities tend to be white male dominated (Garnets and Kimmel, 1991). Moreover, researchers have documented the negative effects of the underrepresentation of GALOCs in positions of power in the gay and lesbian community (Icard, 1986). The unchecked power and privilege of the white gay and lesbian community to dictate gay and lesbian community experience and institutions has led to racial discrimination toward GALOCs.

Discrimination has taken many forms. For example, Asian Americans report being stereotyped as "erotic" or simply remain unacknowledged, invisible, or sexually "neutered" in the gay and lesbian community (Chan, 1989). Similar to Asian Americans, African Americans, Latinos/as, and American Indians also have had to contend with being romanticized, objectified, and eroticized (Icard, 1986; Jaimes and Halsey, 1992). Greene (1993) describes this objectification process of GALOCs by white gays and lesbians as "ethnosexual stereotyping." She identifies ethnosexual stereotyping as the combination of racism and sexism as manifested in the sexual objectification of lesbians and gay men of color according to racial stereotypes (e.g., Asian men as geishas or African men depicted pictorially as huge, muscular men in chains in gay magazines). Moreover, she highlights the need for practitioners to be aware of how GALOCs might internalize the ethnosexual stereotype of their own ethnic group.

Racism is further demonstrated in the discrimination toward GALOCs in admittance to gay bars (e.g., having to provide two or more pieces of identification to get into bars compared to a white, gay counterpart where one or no identification is requested [Icard, 1986]). Moreover, dealing with invisibility in gay and lesbian community settings via being ignored at gay and lesbian social events (Chan, 1989; Greene, 1993) leads to considerable feelings of social isolation and disempowerment.

Among white lesbians, Allman (1996) notes that there is generally an assumption of "normative whiteness" within the term "lesbian." This is similar to the term "American" being implicitly reserved for white Americans or others who are expected to conform or assimilate to white American values and identity. For example, at many lesbian events the term "lesbian" is reserved for white lesbians, as evidenced by book readings by "lesbians" versus book readings by women of color or "lesbians of color." Moreover, Allman (1996, p. 288) notes that "lesbian events may completely ignore nonwhite or mixed-race lesbians or selectively use our perspectives only as they support a 'normative' white lesbian experience or agenda."

In sum, although GALOCs may experience, to some degree, much needed gay and lesbian community support and refuge from societal heterosexism, the strength of that support and the stressors associated with racism diminish the full range of support for GALOCs that is otherwise available to white gays and lesbians. The primary conflict in allegiance that arises as the result of racism in the white gay and lesbian community structure is whether it is worth jeopardizing ethnic community priorities and ties to connect with a community that is wrought with racism. Although there is tremendous need for support to deal with the heterosexism in one's own community of color, the potential loss of support from one's own ethnic community is a price that is too precious to pay for many GALOCs who seek refuge in their own ethnic community to combat racist oppression. The stressors associated with picking one community over the other are tremendous.

Heterosexism in Communities of Color

In addition to being discriminated against by the gay and lesbian community, GALOCs similarly experience rejection, stigmatization, and heterosexism within their own communities of color. However, even though the process parallels the discrimination of white gays and lesbians toward GALOCs, it is not to be mistaken for the same process. The within-group prejudices must be understood as manifestations of internalized, colonized processes within a system of white heterosexual institutionalized systems of power. In other words, the group that ultimately benefits from within-group oppressions is white heterosexual men and to some degree white heterosexual women. Thus, white gays and lesbians reinforce their power as members of white society by being racist, whereas heterosexuals of color do not benefit communities of color by being heterosexist. Having said this, I will explore further the stressors associated with the within-group oppressions among communities of color.

First, GALOCs frequently face questioning of their racial identity if they openly identify as gay or lesbian, since such open identification is at times interpreted as an abandonment of priorities in fighting racial or cultural oppression. For example, Moraga (1983), a mixed Chicana lesbian, states that she has been accused of contributing to the genocide of the Chicano people through her resistance to succumb to cultural gender roles. Thus, for lesbians of color, the interlocking oppressions of heterosexism and sexism may be used by one's community of color as a form of social control (to maintain the illusion of unity) in the fight against racism.

Second, expectations regarding expected cultural gender roles in the continuance and survival of one's race play a critical role in exacerbating conflicts in allegiances for GALOCs. For example, Wong (1992) noted that for Chinese-born American immigrants, compulsory heterosexual relationships in the new country symbolizes a healthy adjustment to the United States. Additionally, displays of assertiveness (sexual or otherwise) in Chinese women are interpreted as emasculating to Chinese men and an assimilation to "unnatural" power imbalances between men and women (Wong, 1992). Thus, any deviation from cultural gender roles may be interpreted as an attack on the group's survival. Such a burden creates considerable stress and conflict for GALOCs.

Lesbians of color face tremendous pressure since both the child-rearing and childbearing roles are closely associated with the culture's continuity and survival. For example, the interactive effects of heterosexism, sexism, and racism for African-American women are demonstrated in the misinterpretation of the strength of African-American women as emasculating to African-American men. Greene (1993) notes that group internalization of such controlling images misnames African-American male oppression as the result of emasculating African-American women, as opposed to the external racist institutions. Such group internalizations structure sexist and heterosexist gender role expectations as commensurate with group survival (Greene, 1993). Pharr (1988) argues that the intersection of heterosexism (including compulsory heterosexuality), sexism, and racism work simultaneously to reinforce racist gender roles. Moreover, these heterocentric, sexist gender roles function as forms of social control to establish group conformity to a unilateral definition of oppressed group membership and group survival. Patricia Hill Collins refers to these socially constructed images or illusions as "controlling images," which serve to reinforce the status quo both within and between groups. Moreover, the implicit assumption inherent in such imperatives is that GALOCs would have no interest in community survival since being gay or lesbian is [mis]associated with the rejection of childbearing or child-rearing roles. Such assumptions are simply unwarranted given that child bearing/rearing and being gay or lesbian are not mutually exclusive states of being (Greene, 1994). Nevertheless, the community internalization of such imperatives creates tremendous stress for GALOCs. Additionally, the GALOC's internalization of such assumptions exacerbates anxiety and feelings of inauthenticity.

GALOCs face additional criticism from their communities of color regarding the notion that homosexuality is a white problem or a pathological response to white racism. Moreover, heterosexual persons of color tend to see identification with another oppressed group as being an unnecessary burden on an already oppressed status. Hemphill (1992), the late African-American activist, asserts that communities of color need to contest black nationalist proclamations that homosexuality is evidence of white inferiority or that black homosexuality is the result of internalized racism. Hemphill argues that communities of color must defy linking compulsory heterosexuality, heterocentricity, or heterosexism with group survival or the battle against racist oppression.

Finally, the issue of visibility also creates tremendous stress for GALOCs. GALOCs frequently receive double-bind messages from their families. GALOCs who choose to be visible or open are subject to having their loyalty to family/community questioned. However, homosexuality might be tolerated by the family or the community as long as it is not visible or spoken of. For example, in a study of thirteen Japanese gay men, Wooden, Kawaksaki, and Mayeda (1983) found that the respondents were primarily concerned about the potential loss and rejection by the Japanese community for being visibly active in the gay community. Other racial groups as well have documented their hesitancy to be open and visible in the gay and lesbian community for fear of the loss of important cultural support systems, rejection from their families, and ultimately, rejection from the community of color at large (Garnets and Kimmel, 1991; Loicano, 1989). For example, studies have shown that African-American lesbians more than white lesbians maintain strong family ties and depend on family for social, emotional, and financial support (Bell and Wienberg, 1978; Croom, 1993; Greene, 1993). The threat of loss or rejection of cultural support leaves GALOCs vulnerable, particularly since family and extended kin networks typically function as the primary refuge against racist oppression (Greene, 1993).

CONCLUSION

The Functions of Heterosexism, Sexism, and Racism

The function of the use and abuse of such controlling images is rooted in sexism, heterosexism, and racism for GALOCs and function as a form of social control for unilateral oppressed-group conformity. These controlling images (Collins, 1990) by both groups (heterosexuals of color and white gay men and lesbians) function to constrain the GALOC's options and to "perpetuate misinformation, and render invisible or exceptional those [GALOCs] that do not fit the negative controlling image" (Allman, 1996). The intersection of sexism and heterosexism within heterosexual communities of color and the intersection of racism and sexism from white gay communities both utilize these controlling images to keep the "other" part of the GALOC's self silenced. Thus, gender and racial role expectations become boundaried by racial, gender, and heterosexual group mandates between and within groups (Allman, 1996), and conflicts in allegiances arise as a response to these life stressors.

As a result of the multiple conflicts in allegiances, many GALOCs feel that they do not completely belong to one group or the other, thereby creating difficulty in consolidating an identity as a

GALOC. Research results have yielded contradictory findings concerning which group the GALOC feels most comfortable with and with which group GALOCs most strongly identify. Espin (1987) noted that Latina lesbians identified with a white lesbian community in one sample. Chan (1989) noted that Asian lesbians identification varied depending on the needs of the individual and the context of the situation. However, many researchers have documented the preference of GALOCs to be accepted and acknowledged by both their ethnic communities and the gay and lesbian community. Nevertheless, achieving this integration has been difficult given the life stressors discussed earlier (Chan, 1989; Espin, 1987; Garnets and Kimmel, 1991).

There is one note of caution in interpreting research results regarding which group GALOCs feel most comfortable with and with which group GALOCs most strongly identify: The majority of GALOC studies are based on self-identified gay men of color and do not always include men who have sex with men who do not identify as gay, bisexual men of color, or gay men who do not openly self-identify among their heterosexual communities of color. As a result, the perception of discrimination on the basis of race or sexual orientation or their strength of persons of color in identification with one community over the other may vary for these other groups.

Despite research shortcomings, many researchers state that for many GALOCs, the ability not to "split" themselves into disparate social parts depends on the situational context, the safety of the situation (ranging from potential physical harm to potential emotional rejection and loss), and the strength of their positive GALOC identity attitudes (Walters, 1997).

The Galoc Identity Matrix Model

In developing a model of GALOC's identity processes, it is important to note that this model is to be used as an initial assessment framework that is modifiable according to the cultural orientation of the individual. Additionally, the GALOC identity matrix provides an initial assessment of potential areas of strength for further reinforcement and areas of vulnerability in need of possible intervention. Based on previous mental health research on GALOC identity models, it is presumed here that by identifying the self and group identity attitudes across racial and homosexual dimensions, the practitioner is better equipped to identify and anticipate problem areas for the GALOC client in negotiating successfully their conflicts in allegiances.

First, GALOCs may be highly ethnically identified and highly gay identified simultaneously, although the two are not necessarily correlated (Walters, 1997). As Oetting and Beauvais (1990-1991) point out, cultural identification is an orthogonal process where identification with one culture does not necessarily mean a lesser identification with another culture. Thus, cultural identification consists of independent identities (gay/lesbian and racial) where individuals can have a unicultural, bicultural, or multicultural identification simultaneously (Walters, 1997).

To facilitate a visual understanding of the GALOC identify matrix model, see Figure 3.1 and Figure 3.2. Although the 2x2 identity matrix is identical for both self and group identity attitudes, both matrices are included here, given the multidimensional complexity. Additionally, since the practitioner needs to assess both group and self identity attitudes, the matrices allow one to visually see the strengths and vulnerabilities that the GALOC individual possesses across both dimensions (racial and sexual orientation attitudes) simultaneously.

As evidenced in Figures 3.1 and 3.2, the GALOC identity matrix embodies two processes. The GALOC's group racial identity attitudes may be high (e.g., positive attitudes toward one's racial group) or low (negative attitudes toward one's racial group) and GALOC gay/lesbian group identity attitudes may be high (e.g., positive attitudes toward gays or lesbians as a group) or low (negative attitudes toward gays or lesbians as a group) on either continuum simultaneously. Additionally, GALOC self identity attitudes may be high (e.g., positive attitudes toward oneself as a person of color) or low (negative attitudes toward oneself as a person of color), and gay/lesbian self-identity attitudes may be high (e.g., positive attitudes toward oneself as a gay or lesbian) or low (negative attitudes toward oneself as a gay or lesbian) on either continuum simultaneously. For example, an African-American lesbian could have positive attitudes toward African-Americans as a group and toward the self as African-American but could hold negative

FIGURE 3.1. *Self Identity* Identity Attitude Matrix for GALOCs

SELF IDENTITY ATTITUDES

Self Identity Attitudes	Gay Positive +	Gay Negative −
Racial Positive +	G+ R+	G − R +
Racial Negative −	G+ R−	G − R −

FIGURE 3.2. *Group Identity* Identity Attitude Matrix for GALOCs

GROUP IDENTITY ATTITUDES

Group Identity Attitudes	Gay Positive +	Gay Negative −
Racial Positive +	G+ R+	G − R +
Racial Negative −	G+ R−	G − R −

attitudes toward gays and lesbians as a group and toward oneself as lesbian. Thus, the GALOC model is also inclusive of the dual dimensionality of the two group identity attitude development processes (racial identity and gay and lesbian group identity) in conjunction with self-identity development (including the stage of coming out to oneself and one's ethnic community).

The level of development in terms of coming out to oneself and to one's ethnic community affects gay and lesbian self and group identity and, therefore, needs to be considered as an added dimension to the GALOC identity matrix model. Ideally, the GALOC individual could have positive attitudes toward being ethnic, toward being a member of the ethnic community, toward being a gay/lesbian person, and toward the gay and lesbian community.

Three Primary Constellations of Identity Matrix Processes for GALOCs

Described below are three primary constellations of racial and sexual orientation attitudinal processes from which the practitioner

can draw inferences about salient assessment and intervention issues facing GALOCs in negotiating their conflicts in allegiances.

Combined Positive Identity Attitudes (G+ R+)

Individuals who possess self and group G+ R+ identity attitudes
are likely to have identity attitudes that buffer against their conflicts
in allegiances, facilitating positive mental health outcomes. Moreover, their GALOC identity attitudes interact with life stressors to
facilitate positive coping responses in successfully negotiating
group tensions. Generally, these individuals will tend to externalize
their conflicts in allegiances, placing the problems of the groups'
heterosexism or racism in proper perspective. Thus, they will likely
be able to confront the heterosexism or racism as an example of
colonized group processes and not internalize it and take inappropriate responsibility for misperceived threats to group survival.
Moreover, GALOCs who have this identity constellation will not
have identity attitudes as a core area for intervention in dealing with
conflicts in allegiances. Rather, the identity attitudes that facilitate
healthy coping will be further strengthened given the GALOC's
social and cultural contexts in which conflicts arise.

Mixed Positive and Negative Identity Attitudes (G+ R- or G- R+)

The individual who presents with self and group G+ R- or G- R+
is at greater risk for difficulties in consolidating a positive GALOC
identity and internalizing colonizing attitudes. The matrix, however,
identifies areas of strength and vulnerability. Thus, if a GALOC
presents with G+ R- identity attitudes, then racial identity functions
as an area for cognitive interventions while it also reinforces the
strengths of the gay or lesbian identity at the same time.

Cognitive interventions and positive reframing are powerful
tools to reconceptualize the conflicts in allegiances as arising from
competing demands of two oppressed groups for group survival.
The key in dealing with this constellation is to assist the GALOC
individual to externalize the internalized group thinking and reframe their experience as not being a threat to group survival.
Additionally, by identifying the R+ or G+ strengths and positive

coping, the GALOC individual can then translate those skills for their R- or G- conflicts. Moreover, it is important to assist GALOCs with identifying and anticipating potential loss or rejection by others in either community. In addition, it is important to strengthen existing support systems that embrace their multiple-situated identities.

Individuals with G+ R- or G- R+ identity attitudes may also experience tremendous emotional ambivalence given the social context, moving from identifying as primarily "gay" in gay settings to primarily "racial" in ethnic community settings, thereby splitting off salient aspects of self given different social contexts. One particular task, given the ambivalence, is to facilitate an integrated identity across multiple settings, although timing of this process is also dependent on the strength and salience of support systems from both communities. Additionally, if the GALOC individual needs to remain as one primary dimension across both settings, then it is important to keep an eye on the potential internalization of colonized group thinking processes and gently challenge them. Finally, individuals in this stage may be most receptive to support groups and contact with other GALOC groups that can facilitate positive integrated role-modeled behaviors for negotiating ongoing conflicts in group allegiances.

Combined Negative Identity Attitudes (G- R-)

GALOC individuals who are self and group G- and R- are the most vulnerable to tremendous difficulty in dealing with group conflicts. Moreover, they are likely to be socially isolated since they hold negative attitudes toward both racial and gay/lesbian groups as well as their own sense of self as an ethnic and gay/lesbian person. As a result, their ability to reconcile multiple life stressors will be compromised since they will not have many group survival skills to assist them in coping with group conflicts. These individuals will tend to minimize their gay or lesbian status and their racial status as significant aspects of their lives (this of course is due to their internalization of negative dominant group attitudes, not their sense of self-group actualization). Moreover, they will try to distance themselves from either group and try to "pass" as "just a person" and identify with a dominant white heterosexual society. They will also hold very negative attitudes toward other gays or lesbians as well as people of color.

GALOCs experiencing both negative self and group identity attitudes will not perceive conflicts in allegiances as a stressor until they are confronted with either coming out to others or they are confronted by members of the gay or lesbian community or their ethnic community regarding their group loyalties. These GALOCs will have tremendous difficulty negotiating multiple levels of internalized negative attitudes about themselves as persons of color who are gay or lesbian.

It is important to focus initially on gently confronting negative stereotypes internalized by the GALOC, facilitating connections with other positive GALOC role models, and anticipating potential loss or rejection by others. Moreover, the primary issue for GALOCs experiencing such conflicts, given this identity matrix constellation, is that they are anticipating a perceived loss or rejection by one community or the other. It is imperative that one assess how the GALOC has coped with loss previously while simultaneously reframing and translating the strengths in previous coping for the current stressor. One form of coping may be to split off the self, given the social context for GALOCs at this stage (similar to individuals possessing mixed positive and negative group and self identity attitudes discussed previously). This may be a necessary first step, but it must be made thoughtfully with the practitioner remaining cognizant of potential internalization of negative group messages. For example, the GALOC may choose to come out to someone from their ethnic community but choose to remain closeted within the larger ethnic community. This can be seen as an important step toward integration and consolidation of self and group identity.

Although these three primary constellations are not exhaustive (there are sixteen possible combinations of self and group identity racial and gay/lesbian identity attitudes that are beyond the scope of this chapter), the practitioner can utilize the above matrices to identify areas of strength and vulnerability in assessing GALOC identity attitudes and GALOCs' coping abilities in negotiating the conflicts in allegiances. Moreover, the matrices will highlight how the identity attitudes may be moderating the effects of conflicting allegiances on psychological wellness. For example, if one has both negative self and group GALOC identity attitudes, then the practitioner can identify the ways in which these identity attitudes effectively and negatively interact with the GALOC's conflicts in allegiances and their corresponding anxiety or depression (i.e., mental health outcomes).

It is important to keep in mind that GALOCs may pass through different combinations of self and group identity attitudes throughout their lifetime and may "spiral" back through earlier constellations at higher levels, experiencing early constellation/matrix traits if external impingements and sociohistorical circumstances exacerbate life stressors and increase feelings of isolation and powerlessness (Walters and Simoni, 1993).

Social Work Practice Issues

In addition to the assessment of the client's identity attitude matrix, the GALOC client's experience of stressors associated with acculturation, cultural value conflicts, and immigration status must also be assessed. These four factors (identity attitudes, acculturation level, cultural values, and immigration status) help the social work practitioner identify areas of vulnerability in need of intervention and strengthening.

Acculturative Stress

Cultural Values and Conflicts

Several empirical studies are now beginning to suggest that one could be highly acculturated while simultaneously being highly ethnically identified and vice-versa (Hutnik, 1985; Kemnitzer, 1978; Zak, 1976). However, despite the promise of research highlighting the multidimensionality of acculturation processes, many GALOCs, like other oppressed populations, experience intense pressure to relinquish their own ethnic community cultural values and replace them with the dominant (in this case, white gay and lesbian community values) culture's values. For GALOCS, the acculturative stress that results from the pressures to acculturate is manifested in the assumptions from the gay and lesbian community's cultural value to "come out" to others as a mental health and political imperative. However, for many GALOCs "coming out" may at times conflict with their own cultural values. For example, among some American Indian populations, coming out is a value that is dissonant with the cultural value of anonymity, where drawing attention to one's own needs is contrary to the collectivist nature of the culture. The individualism implicit in coming out may be seen as an affront to the higher order value (in some cultures) placed on the sense of self in relation to the collective (see Walters, 1997 for further details).

Another acculturative stressor that GALOCs must contend with is the different acculturation levels of their families and community-kin networks in relation to their own acculturation levels. Any difference in acculturation levels creates further stress regarding reconciling one's own values and the values of one's culture and family. Thus, GALOC assessment should also identify the cultural values that are still held intact by the GALOC and his or her kin networks. This includes words and phrases regarding gay or lesbians in the culture of the GALOC and the meaning of being gay or lesbian from the cultural perspective (Espin, 1987). For example, identifying traditional ways in which GALOCs have a role that is specific to his or her culture may be helpful (especially for two-spirit or gay/lesbian American Indians [Walters, 1996]). Moreover, the worker should assess the possibility of incorporating other members of the clients' family network, GALOC culture-specific community members, or traditional healers/medicine persons to help the client integrate a positive GALOC identity (Walters, 1997).

Ultimately, acculturative stress may affect GALOCs' attitudes toward identifying with other GALOCs. For example, if an assimilationist ideology is internalized within a particular cultural group and is rooted in heterocentric biases from the dominant society, then the probability for contacting other GALOCs from one's own culture is diminished. Additionally, there is an increased chance of isolation (Berry, Kim, Minde, and Mok, 1987; Cornell, 1988; Kraus and Buffler, 1979) from important GALOC cultural supports, positive within-group GALOC role models, and GALOC survival strategies.

To deal with conflicting allegiances associated with acculturative stress, LaFromboise (1988) and Moncher, Holden, and Trimble

(1990) advocate development of a "bicultural competence reper-toire." They state that such a repertoire assists Indian youth in developing adaptive coping responses to the interaction between their tribal culture and that of the majority culture. Similarly, GA-LOCs could benefit from developing a bicultural competence reper-toire in assisting them in successfully negotiating conflicts in alle-giances—both between groups (i.e., with white gays and lesbian communities) and within groups (i.e., different acculturation levels across self, family, and kin networks). For example, GALOC bicul-tural competence would assist GALOCs in integrating positive as-pects of both cultures (gay/lesbian and racial/cultural) without los-ing their own cultural values or internalizing heterosexist biases.

Immigration Issues

Immigration status also is a critical factor in affecting the GA-LOC's successful negotiation of conflicts in allegiances. Espin (1987) notes that the time and reasons for immigrating to the United States are factors in shaping how GALOCs perceive and experience conflicts in allegiances. For example, even though immigration might be voluntary, GALOCs still experience significant losses of familial support systems upon arrival to the United States, even if they were leaving their country of origin to seek a more gay-affirmative environment. Additionally, if immigration is recent, the GALOC might lose significant economic support from his or her family and become dependent on extended family in the U.S. or on other ethnic community members (Espin, 1987). The interdepen-dence on ethnic community financial and emotional supports makes it even more difficult to come out to one's ethnic community or consolidate one's multiple-situated identities (Greene, 1993).

In sum, level of acculturation (including the generation level) and corresponding acculturative stress, immigration status, and in-ternalization of cultural values and frameworks are important fac-tors that must be incorporated into GALOC assessment. They can provide information as to the appropriate areas of intervention, whether it is within the individual in terms of helping the GALOC client integrate both identities or whether it is external (i.e., fighting heterosexism or racism at the community level [Walters, 1996]).

Social Work Practice Skills

Empowerment-Oriented Reframing

In line with the ecological model of practice (Germain and Gitterman, 1996), a positive reframe of the stressors associated with multiple-situated identities assists GALOCs with negotiating a "border" status (Anzaldua, 1987). Anzaldua suggests that multiple-status individuals can bridge both communities by having both feet solidly planted in both worlds. This positive reframe suggests that GALOCs have the right to not fractionalize their allegiances and can integrate multiple perspectives and statuses simultaneously (Anzaldua, 1987; Root, 1996; Williams, 1996). Anzaldua states that to develop a new "border" consciousness we need to affirm the marginalized parts of self (whether racial, gender, or sexual orientation) and integrate them–to heal the conflicts in allegiances within one's self. This act reflects healthy resistance to internalized oppression.

Another opportunity for a positive reframe is to challenge the notion that to be a GALOC means that one is "caught" or "stuck" between worlds and communities. As a practitioner, one can reframe this intermediary position not as a problem, but, rather, as an opportunity to have a unique vantage point, from which an analysis of conflicting allegiances, GALOC marginalization, and assumptions of community legitimacy are possible (Kich, 1996; hooks, 1981). Kich notes that "both insider and outsider positions can be reframed as a source of positive learning for marginalized peoples" (p. 271). Thus, the task for the practitioner is to reframe the marginalization (which is the result of the internalization of group imperatives rooted in heterosexism, racism, and sexism) as an opportunity to achieve new insight into the assumptions of community legitimacy and ultimately challenge such assumptions when they are oppressive to community members (Kich, 1996). By embracing the position of a multiple-situated identity, GALOCs can challenge the status quo of both the gay and lesbian community and their respective communities of color.

Assisting GALOCs with positive reframing of the conflicts in allegiances that naturally arise when oppressed groups attempt to survive requires considerable cognitive flexibility on both the practitioner's and client's parts. Cognitive flexibility (i.e., the ability to integrate both categories as salient and noncompetitive [Kich, 1996]) is the hallmark of multicultural social work practice. Kich (1996, p. 275) states that "a person's degree of emotional/cognitive/social flexibility [the ability to tolerate and to manage increased levels of complexity and differentiation] may be understood as a developmental consequence of a healthy adaptation to life."

Another intervention includes helping the client to find culturally relevant ways to "come out" that do not deny or split off the gay or lesbian or ethnic aspect of self. If the problems of the GALOC client are less internal (i.e., the client is coping fairly well) and are more external (i.e., due to heterosexism or racism) then identifying ways to educate others or to employ social action strategies to confront such oppression can be explored as well.

Too often a deficit model focusing on the negatives in identity development among oppressed groups has dominated mental health approaches to direct practice. To counter this, social work practitioners need to focus on the GALOC's resilience and positive coping. Focusing on resilience will help to counter the difficulty in dealing with a disparaged status in a society that oppresses persons of color and gays and lesbians. Additionally, by focusing on a GALOC client's strengths, the practitioner reminds the GALOC client of his or her sources of strength and reinforces a positive sense of an integrated self (Walters, 1997).

Mezzo and Macro Levels of Practice

Dispelling stereotypes and providing access to positive GALOC role models that are culturally specific to the GALOC's culture are important community, family, and individual interventions (Walters, 1997). Panel presentations that include GALOC role models are particularly helpful in changing community attitudes. In terms of the gay and lesbian community, GALOC panel presentations address issues of invisibility and racism in gay and lesbian communities. For communities of color, GALOC panels or panelists debunk within-group stereotypes, heterosexism, and group denial of GALOC existence. On the individual level, GALOC involvement in more gay and/or ethnic community contacts may be an appropriate intervention if one or the other identity is neglected due to the conflicts in allegiances that are identified in the GALOC identity attitudes matrix model.

Social work practitioners should be aware of the interplay between intrapsychic problems and external, systemic factors such as heterosexism and racism in individual GALOC functioning and in community functioning (Walters, 1996; Walters and Simoni, 1993). Practitioner effectiveness will be dependent on the ability to differentiate among these systemic factors (Trimble, 1981; Trimble and LaFromboise, 1985). Understanding the multidimensionality of the GALOC experience and the corresponding factors that contribute to identity attitude development; maintenance of within-group heterosexism, racism, and sexism; and the resulting conflicts in allegiances assists practitioners and program planners in developing culturally relevant treatment strategies and agency programs (Walters, 1997). By better understanding the complexities of within- and between-group pressures that GALOC's face, administrators and practitioners may be able to identify preference for a gay clinician, a nongay practitioner of color, or a practitioner who is also a GALOC (depending on the levels of GALOC identity attitudes [Walters, 1997]).

In terms of community-oriented empowerment practice, heterosexual communities of color and white gay and lesbian communities must first recognize their role in marginalizing GALOCs. When members of one group intimidate others within their own group, their marginalizing power ultimately undermines group unity to fight oppression.

Additionally, community-based practice involves mild confrontation regarding racist and heterosexist community norms. One way to challenge community racism and heterosexism is to develop community relational competence (Kich, 1996). According to Kich relational competence is defined as the "interest and capacity to stay emotionally present with, to enlarge or deepen the relational context to create enough 'space' for both or all people to express themselves, and to allow for possible conflict, tension and creative resolution" (p. 275). Flexibility of constructs, relational competence, and adaptability are the community-based social skills to living with difference, without creating conflicts in allegiances within and between communities and, ultimately, within and between the GALOC's sense of self.

Future Research

In terms of future research, the role of religion in GALOC's community life needs to be further explored. Moreover, the GALOC identity attitude matrix model needs to be empirically tested for its psychometric rigor. Additionally, the stress/identity/mental wellness paradigm needs to be empirically tested. Furthermore, the issues men who have sex with men but who do not identify as gay, as well as bisexuals of color, and also biracial or multiracial GALOCs need to be examined in future discussions.

In sum, Audre Lorde (1984) reminds us that in order to support healthy, integrated GALOC individuals and communities, we must recognize multiple identities and allegiances, examine multiple and simultaneous oppressions, and dismantle within- and between-group oppressive hierarchies.

REFERENCES

Allman, K. M. (1996). (Un)Natural boundaries: Mixed race, gender, and sexuality. In M. P. P. Root (Ed.), *The multiracial experience: Racial borders as the new frontier* (pp. 275-290). Thousand Oaks, CA: Sage Publisher.

Anzaldua, G. (1987). *Borderlands/LaFrontera: The new Mestiza.* San Francisco: Spinsters/Aunt Lute Foundation.

Atkinson, D., Morten, G., and Sue, D. (1983). *Counseling American minorities.* Dubuque, ID: W. C. Brown.

Bell, A. and Weinberg, M. (1978). *Homosexualities: A study of human diversity among men and women.* New York: Simon and Schuster.

Berry, J., Kim, U., Minde, T., and Mok, D. (1987). Comparative studies of acculturative stress. *International Migration Review, 21,* 491-511.

Cass, V. C. (1984). Homosexual identity formation: Testing a theoretical model. *Journal of Sex Research, 20,* 143-167.

Chan, C. (1989). Issues of identity development among Asian-American lesbians and gay men. *Journal of Counseling and Development, 68*(1), 16-20.

Collins, P. H. (1990). Homophobia and black lesbians. In *Black feminist thought: Knowledge, consciousness, and the politics of empowerment* (pp. 192-196). Boston: Unwin Hyman.

Cornell, S. (1988). The transformations of tribe: Organization and self-concept in Native American ethnicities. *Ethnic and Racial Studies, 11,* 27-47.

Croom, G. (1993). *The effects of a consolidated versus non-consolidated identity on expectations of African-American lesbians selecting mates: A pilot study.* Unpublished doctoral dissertation, Illinois School of Professional Psychology, Chicago, IL.

Cross, W. (1978). The Thomas and Cross models of psychological nigrescence: A literature review. *Journal of Black Psychology, 4,* 13-31.

Dinges, N. G. and Joos, S. K., (1988). *Stress, coping, and health: Models of interaction for Indian and Native populations in behavioral health issues among American Indians and Alaska Natives,* Vol. 1, 8-64.

Dohrenwend, B. S. and Dohrenwend, B. P. (Eds.). (1981). *Stressful life events and their contexts.* New York: Neale Watson Academic Publications.

Espin, O. (1987). Issues of identity in the psychology of Latina lesbians. In Boston Lesbian Psychologies Collective (Ed.), *Lesbian psychologies: Explorations and challenges* (pp.35-51). Urbana, IL: University of Illinois Press.

Garnets, L. and Kimmel, D. (1991). Lesbian and gay male dimensions in the psychological study of human diversity. In J. D. Goodchilds (Ed.), *Psychological perspectives on human diversity: Master lecturer series* (pp. 143-189). Washington, DC: American Psychological Association.

Germain, C. B. and Gitterman, A. (1996). *The life model of social work practice: Advances in theory and practice,* (second edition). New York: Columbia University Press.

Greene, B. (1993). Stereotypes of African American sexuality: A commentary. In S. Rathus, J. Nevid, and L. Rathus-Fichner (Eds.), *Human sexuality in a world of diversity* (p. 257). Boston: Allyn and Bacon.

Greene, B. (1994). Lesbian women of color: Triple jeopardy. In Comas-Diaz, L., and Greene, B. (Eds.), *Women of color: Integrating ethnic and gender identities in psychotherapy* (pp. 339-427). New York: The Guilford Press.

Helms, J. E. (1989). Considering some methodological issues in racial identity research. *The Counseling Psychologist, 17*(2), 227-252.

Helms, J. (1990). *Black and White racial identity attitudes: Theory, practice, and research.* New York: Greenwood Press.

Hemphill, E. (1992). *Ceremonies: Prose and poetry.* New York: Plume/Penguin.

Hendin, H. (1969). *Black suicide.* New York: Basic Books.

hooks, b. (1981). *Ain't I a woman: Black women and feminism.* Boston: South End Press.

Hutnik, N. (1985). Aspects of identity in a multi-ethnic society. *New Community, 12,* 298-309.

Icard, L. (1986). Black gay men and conflicting social identities: Sexual orientation versus racial identity. In J. Gripton and M. Valentich (Eds.), *Journal of Social Work and Human Sexuality: Social Work Practice in Sexual Problems* [Special Issue], *4*(1/2), 83-93.

Jaimes, M. A. and Halsey, T. (1992). American Indian women: At the center of indigenous resistance in North America. In M. A. Jaimes (Ed.), *The state of Native America: Genocide, colonization, and resistance* (pp. 311-344). Boston: South End Press.

Johnson, J. (1982). *The influence of assimilation on the psychosocial adjustment of black homosexual men.* Unpublished dissertation, California School of Professional Psychology, Berkeley, California.

Kemnitzer, L. S. (1978). Adjustment and value conflict in urbanizing Dakota Indians measured by Q-Sort technique. *American Anthropologist, 75,* 687-707.

Kich, G. K. (1996). In the margins of sex and race: Difference, marginality, and flexibility. In M. P. P. Root, (Ed.), *The multiracial experience: Racial borders as the new frontier* (pp. 263-274). Thousand Oaks, CA: Sage Publisher.

Kraus, R. F. and Buffler, P. A. (1979). Sociocultural stress and the American Native in Alaska: An analysis of changing patterns of psychiatric illness and alcohol abuse among Alaska Natives. *Culture, Medicine and Psychiatry, 3,* 111-151.

LaFromboise, T. D. (1988). American Indian mental health policy. *American Psychologist, 43,* 388-397.

Lazarus, R. (1980). The stress and coping paradigm. In L. Bond and J. Rosen, (Eds.), *Competence and coping during adulthood* (pp. 28-74). Hanover, NH: University Press of New England.

Loiacano, D. K. (1989). Gay identity issues among Black Americans: Racism, homophobia, and the need for validation. *Journal of Counseling and Development, 68,* 21-25.

Lorde, A. (1984). Our difference is our strength. *MS. Magazine* (1996), Vol. VII, (1), 61-64. Reprinted from Age, race, class, and sex: Women redefining difference. In A. Lorde, *Sister outsider.* Freedom, CA: The Crossing Press.

Moncher, M., Holden, G. W., and Trimble, J. E. (1990). Substance abuse among Native American youth. *Journal of Consulting and Clinical Psychology, 58,* 408-415.

Moraga, C. (1983). *Loving in the war years.* Boston: South End Press.

Morales, E. S. (1989). Ethnic minority families and minority gays and lesbians. *Marriage and Family Review, 14,* 217-239.

Oetting, E. R., and Beauvais, F. (1990-1991). Orthogonal cultural identification theory: The cultural identification of minority adolescents. *The International Journal of the Addictions, 25,* (5A, 6A), 655-685.

Parham, T. and Helms, J. (1985a). Attitudes of racial identity and self-esteem of black students: An exploratory investigation. *Journal of College Student Personnel, 26,* 143-147.

Parham, T. and Helms, J. (1985b). Relation of racial identity attitudes to self-actualization and affective states of black students. *Journal of Counseling Psychology, 32,* 431-440.

Pharr, S. (1988). *Homophobia: A weapon of sexism.* Little Rock, AR: Chardon Press.

Phinney, J. (1990). Ethnic identity in adolescents and adults: Review of research. *Psychological Bulletin, 108*(3), 499-514.

Root, M. P. P. (1996). (Ed.). *The multiracial experience: Racial borders as the new frontier.* Thousand Oaks, CA: Sage Publisher.

Sue, S. (1992). Ethnicity and culture in psychological research and practice. In J. D. Goodchilds (Ed.), *Psychological perspectives on human diversity in America: Master lecture Series* (pp. 51-85). Washington, DC: American Psychological Association.

Trimble, J. E. (1981). Value differentials and their importance in counseling American Indians. In P. B. Pederson, J. G. Draguns, W. J. Lonner, and J. E. Trimble (Eds.), *Counseling across cultures.* Honolulu: University of Hawaii Press.

Trimble, J. E. and LaFromboise, T. (1985). American Indians and the counseling process: Culture, adaptation, and style. In P. B. Pederson (Ed.), *Handbook of cross-cultural counseling and therapy,* 127-134. Westport, CT: Greenwood Press.

Walters, K. L. (1995). *Urban American Indian identity and psychological wellness.* Unpublished doctoral dissertation, University of California, Los Angeles.

Walters, K. L. (1997). Urban lesbian and gay American Indian identity: Implications for mental health social service delivery. *Journal of Gay and Lesbian Social Services, 6(2)*

Walters, K. L. and Simoni, J. M. (1993). Lesbian and gay male group identity attitudes and self-esteem: Implications for counseling. *The Journal of Counseling Psychology, 40,* 94-99.

Williams, T. K. (1996). Race as process: Reassessing the "What are You" encounters of biracial individuals. In the margins of sex and race: Difference, marginality, and flexibility. In M. P. P. Root, (Ed.), *The multiracial experience: Racial borders as the new frontier* (pp.191-210). Thousand Oaks, CA: Sage Publisher.

Wooden, W. S., Kawaksaki, H., and Mayeda, R. (1983). Lifestyles and identity maintenance among gay Japanese-American males. *Alternative Lifestyles, 5,* 236-243.

Wong, S. C. (1992). Ethnicizing gender, gendering ethnicity. In S. G. Lim and A. Ling (Eds.), *Reading the literatures of Asian America* (pp. 111-129). Philadelphia: Temple University Press.

Zak, I. (1976). Structure of ethnic identity of Arab-Israeli students. *Psychological Reports, 38,* 239-246.

Chapter 4

Individual Practice with Gay Men

Michael Shernoff

INTRODUCTION

Social workers preparing to do individual practice with men who identify as gay need to understand that these clients will present at any social service or health care agency or in private practice seeking direct or clinical social work services. These men may be at any stage of the life cycle, and it is crucial that social workers do not make any assumptions about the nature of these clients or their presenting problems prior to doing a complete psychosocial assessment. In addition, it is important for social workers to understand that men who simply have sex with other men, repeatedly and over time, may never identify themselves as homosexual or gay (Kinsey, Pomeroy, and Martin, 1948). Thus, in order to successfully intervene with this population, social workers should familiarize themselves with the various stages of gay identity formation that homosexually active men may be at in the process of forming an identity as a gay man (Cass, 1979; Coleman, 1988; Isay, 1989).

Germain (1981) and Gitterman and Germain (1976) both discuss social work practice in terms of both understanding and being able to intervene on both the ecological or environmental level as well as with the individual client and his or her immediate system. Germain (1980) explains that "ecology seeks to understand the transactions that take place between environments and living systems and the consequence of these transactions for each." She also elaborates on how an ecological perspective is a useful lens through which to examine the social context of clinical social work. It is essential for the social worker to incorporate an ecological perspective into his or her clinical work with clients from any marginalized population like racial, ethnic, or sexual minorities. It is only through utilizing this broad systems perspective that a worker will be able to understand and correctly reflect back to the client how the biases and assumptions of the mainstream culture have impacted them and contributed to their unique psychodynamic and psychosocial realities. In the case of gay men, this means that an awareness on the worker's part about how the pervasiveness of both societal and internalized homophobia, as well as heterosexual bias, has affected the client's development, self-image, and current functioning, both adaptively and maladaptively. The material in this chapter is based on over twenty years of direct clinical practice with gay men, initially in agency work and private practice, and since 1983, exclusively in private practice. Additionally, the author draws on experiences from supervising clinical social workers in practice with gay men.

DEFINITION

Gonsiorek and Rudolph (1991) state that developing a gay identity would be highly sensitive to cultural, class, socioeconomic, racial, and ethnic variation. Economic privilege provides middle class gay men with opportunities to experiment with forming gay identities—opportunities that are lacking for men who must continue to live with families and rely upon them for concrete support. Therefore, one area that will be tremendously useful for any social worker seeking to provide services to gay men is to develop cultural competency in order to have the sensitivity and skills necessary to work with men who come from various racial, cultural, religious, and economic backgrounds.

It is a mistake to make assumptions about who is and who is not gay simply on the basis of appearances. A client may in fact be gay but look and initially present as indistinguishable from a heterosexual man. Many men who have a current self-definition as gay have gone through periods of their lives when they attempted to hide their homosexual feelings from themselves and others, some marrying and fathering children (Ross, 1983). Other men choose to remain married even after accepting their homosexual feelings (Wyers, 1987). With increasing frequency, openly gay men are choosing to adopt or actually father and raise children (Martin, 1993; Shernoff, 1996). There are times that these men are reluctant to seek out services from openly gay clinicians out of fear of being pressured into coming out or ending long-term marriages to women. Ultimately, the only time a worker knows with certainty that a client is gay is when and if he chooses to disclose his sexual orientation. It is never the goal of treatment to make the client feel that he must reveal his sexual orientation, but rather that the worker can tolerate his or her own discomfort with the client's unwillingness to label where he may be on the spectrum of sexual orientation.

Social workers need to be prepared to work with some heterosexually married male clients who are sexually active and even romantically involved with other men. Counseling these men is complex, and the clients will be alert to any indications of being judged by the worker. Bozett (1981) points out that these men often experience difficulty in achieving a positive gay identity in part because of the perceived incongruity between the two identities of father and gay man. When a heterosexually married, but homosexually active man is HIV seropositive or has AIDS, there are potentially complicated legal and ethical questions for the clinician if the client has not disclosed his health status to his wife.

Wyers (1987) posits that formerly married gay men are likely to fall into two different groups. When the men have not fully acknowledged to themselves or to others that they are homosexual, the services they require are similar to the services needed by other gay men who are in the early process of coming out. After resolving some or many of their personal problems with being homosexual, they may need assistance in working out relationships and custody issues with their former spouses and children. Concerns about custody of or at least access to children is of prime importance to gay fathers. When a gay man has children who live with him at least part time, family therapy is very useful, especially if the client resides with a male lover and stepparenting concerns need to be addressed (Shernoff, 1984).

ASSESSMENT

Gay men who seek social work services manifest all the symptoms and present the same variety of problems as do every other kind of client. In addition, they often have some unique issues arising from their sexual orientation, including adaptation to their current stage of gay identity formation (Cass, 1979, Coleman, 1988); the impact of homophobia, which is defined as the "negative attitudes toward homosexual persons and homosexuality" (Herek, 1990, p. 552); social stigma; a sense of isolation and alienation; coming out; rejection by families of origin; being victims of antigay violence; and the impact of AIDS on their own lives and the lives of their friends and lovers. When gay men are economically disadvantaged, their needs for social services such as public assistance, food stamps, Medicare, or housing, take precedence over issues related to sexual orientation.

"The lesbian and gay communities have been living with the traumatic impact of HIV/AIDS for over a decade. Assessments of the coping and adaptation patterns of gay men seeking psychotherapy have to include the effects of trauma." (Mancoske and Lindhorst, 1995, p. 31). The same authors correctly postulate that the paradigm shift from pathology to empowerment of the oppressed is challenged to expand yet again to models of empowerment of the oppressed who are living with ongoing trauma.

In 1973, the American Psychiatric Association ceased to specify homosexual adjustment as psychopathological (Bayer, 1981). The American Psychiatric Association's official position is that " . . . homosexuality itself is not considered a mental disorder" (American Psychiatric Association, 1987). Letters to the editor, in 1993 issues of *NASW News*, the organization's newspaper, which concerned so-called "Reparative Therapy for Gay Men" (and aid in helping them change their sexual orientation) demonstrate that some social workers in North America remain convinced otherwise (Theriot 1993a, Theriot, 1993b). There are still some clinicians who try to change a client's sexual orientation, though there is no evidence that this is possible and there are strong indications that it has a deleterious effect on the client (Davison, 1982; Martin, 1984). Numerous men have arrived in the author's private practice profoundly depressed and/or highly anxious as a direct result of failed psychotherapeutic attempts to change their sexual orientation. These clients need nurturance in the form of helping them understand that there is nothing intrinsically wrong with their sexual orientation, and that society's homophobia and intolerance is the cause of their distress. One way of accomplishing this is through the use of bibliotherapy, where gay affirmative readings are assigned and discussed during sessions. Sometimes just the assignment of going to a lesbian or gay bookstore and having the client browse will be a powerful initial healing intervention when he or she sees so many titles that reflect the diversity of the gay community. Theoretically, this kind of intervention represents the kind of synthesis of both ego-psychology and the ecological social work perspective discussed by Germain (1978).

Smith (1988, p. 62) makes the point that "an understanding of the intrapsychic and psychosocial factors contributing to psychopathology in homosexually oriented persons requires a clear appreciation of the role of homophobia." Since some gay men do manifest psychiatric illness, social workers must be skilled in diagnosing any psychiatric symptoms in order to be most helpful to clients.

Clinical social workers need to be aware that gay men seeking treatment can present with indications of severe anxiety or depression, thought disorder, persistent characterological problems, chemical dependency, neuropsychological impairment, psychosis, etc. These symptoms may be in addition to or instead of issues related to societal oppression and coming out (Gonsiorek, 1982). Gonsiorek writes, "The coming out process by itself can produce in some individuals psychiatric symptomatology that is reminiscent of serious underlying psychopathology" (p. 11). In addition, many high-functioning gay men seek out therapy for help in improving the interpersonal areas of their lives. This takes the form of men who are professionally successful and who have friends, and by all appearances live a self-actualized life but are not happy about the lack of a satisfying primary romantic relationship.

ETHNIC AND CULTURAL DIVERSITY

There are no stereotypes or generalizations that are universally relevant to all gay men. Differences exist in class, ethnicity, health status, rural or urban environment, and stage of gay identity formation. The skilled social worker must assess the impact of the above issues in addition to the individual's psychodynamics, ego strengths, and social supports. For instance, a middle-class, gay, white man who lives in a large city and who does not conceal his sexual orientation from family, friends, colleagues, or employer may view being gay as his primary cultural identification of at least equal importance to his religious or ethnic background. In contrast, a poor, inner-city gay man of color often views his experience of being black or Latino as the primary way he relates to the world and to a social service agency or practitioner even if the presenting problem is somehow associated with his homosexuality.

Commonly, African-American gay men feel torn between loyalties to homophobic black community institutions or families and racist gay white culture (Icard, 1985-1986; Loiacano, 1989). The author's experience has been that successful professional gay African-American men in his practice have reported a significant degree of pain about the lack of acceptance for them as total human beings within either of their two communities. The most self-actualized clients in this category find deep nurturance within the traditional institutions of the African-American community and at the same time have developed a peer support group of other gay men of color, who function as additional family.

Understanding and responding to cultural differences becomes crucial when attempting to intervene with nonwhite gay men around such life-threatening situations as AIDS-prevention efforts. De la Vega (1995) notes that "it is difficult to speak of sexuality issues among Latinos in the U.S. as if they were just one homogeneous group of individuals." The worker must be alert to distinctive differences of clients of various Hispanic nationalities. For instance, a gay man from Argentina will not have many cultural identifications with a Mexican American or a Puerto Rican.

Carballo-Dieguez (1989) points out that when counseling gay Latino men, religion and folk beliefs must be considered. The impact of conservative Catholicism and its emphasis on traditional values (which strongly reject gay love or sexual expression) is a powerful influence for most Latino men. Although gay Latino men will generally refrain from discussing Santeria and Espiritismo (Spiritualism) with non-Latino professionals out of fear that they will not be taken seriously, these widespread folk beliefs should be explored in counseling and therapy with gay Latino men (Baez, 1996; Carballo-Dieguez, 1989).

Similar issues arise when working with Native American gay men. Tafoya and Rowell (1988) write,

> One must remember there is no such thing as "the" American Indian; rather, there are literally hundreds of different tribes with different languages, customs and world views. Native American gay and lesbian clients often combine elements of common gay experiences with the uniqueness of their own ethnicity. To treat them only as gay and to ignore important cultural issues may bring therapy sessions to a quick end with little accomplished. (p. 64)

Chan (1989) explains that for Asian-American gay men identifying as gay may be perceived as a rejection of traditional family roles and Asian cultural values. However, to identify as Asian American may require negating one's gay identity, at least within the family. Therefore Asian-American gay men often develop a dual identity that encompasses both facets of their cultural identification (See also Sullivan, 1995).

RURAL GAY MEN

Little is known about the lives of rural gay men and the barriers they encounter when in need of social services (Gunter, 1988). Moses and Bucker (1980) have identified specific problem areas, such as the clients' isolation, fear of discovery of their homosexuality, and the effects of generalized anxiety on self-image. They go on to address issues that a professional should consider when providing services to rural gay men. These included clients' misconceptions and attitudes about being gay, lack of local resources and information systems, limited options and alternatives, and the need for the worker to assess the situation realistically.

Breeze (1985) discusses the need for legal assistance and networking services in order to intervene effectively with this population. He asserts that the professional must be prepared to become involved in some or all of the following activities in order to work productively with rural gay men: advocacy work, educating professionals and other service providers about problem areas, and actively enlisting support from other sympathetic professionals.

Gunter (1988) cautions against the assumption that the majority of gay men and lesbians are natives of the metropolitan and suburban environments in which they end up living: "Individuals who have successfully adapted to a gay lifestyle within a metropolitan area may have difficulties during visits home or when family and friends visit the city" (p. 50).

In the same article, Gunter explains that confidentiality is a difficult issue in rural communities since many agencies utilize paraprofessionals and volunteers to provide services. There is a legitimate fear on the part of the gay individual seeking services that his or her sexual orientation will be disclosed to other members of a small community, resulting in ostracism or worse. This fear of exposure limits the gay individual's activities and prevents successful identification with other gay people. The rest of this article will focus on individual clinical practice issues relevant to gay men.

DEPRESSION AND DEVELOPMENTAL ISSUES

Chronic, low-grade depression is often the reason gay men seek therapeutic assistance. These symptoms can sometimes arise out of uncompleted developmental stages of gay identity formation in individuals experiencing a conflict between behaviors and values when they are still undisclosed to important people in their lives (Smith, 1988). In other gay men, long-term symptoms of depression are masked by substance abuse and only emerge after the individual begins recovery from chemical dependency. Clinical social workers working with gay men must become skilled in diagnosing depression and urging clients to have consultations with a gay-sensitive psychopharmacologist regarding beginning a treatment regime of antidepressant medication.

For some depressed gay men, therapy needs to facilitate disclosure (when appropriate) and peer socialization. The sense of belonging to a community and the formation of a network of support among friends and family will protect against decompensation during times of stress. A decrease in social isolation, if present, must be a goal in psychotherapy (Smith, 1988).

Germain's (1980) description of an environmental or ecological approach to clinical social work is once again a useful theoretical framework for making appropriate interventions with gay men that are actually within the realm of "milieu therapy" (for example, introducing the concept of "homosocializing" [Isay, 1989] to a client). Often it is appropriate to explore the client's knowledge of gay social organizations and clubs where he or she might go to meet other men who have similar interests. In order to help facilitate the development of relationships with peers, social workers need to be aware of local resources for gay clients and how to direct the client in their direction. Most large cities now have gay political, athletic, social, and religious groups that can provide clients with the opportunity to strengthen affiliations with other gay men.

Many gay men do not accomplish the normal developmental tasks of adolescence, such as forming a peer group, exploring sexuality, experimenting with intimacy and initial forays into love when they are in their teens or their twenties. Therefore, when experiencing some of the turbulence and emotionality of teenagers as adults in their twenties, thirties, or even older, there is a dissonance between chronological age and the developmental tasks they are struggling with. This discrepancy between age and developmental tasks is often the source of high anxiety and/or depression that is resolved as the individual gains mastery over these new situations. Thus there are frequently aspects of psychotherapy with gay men that are in fact counseling rather than intrapsychic explorations of unresolved feelings. Very often the content of therapy sessions will focus on how to learn the various social skills necessary to meet and date other men and similar issues relating to practical concerns like safe sex.

During the course of therapy, most gay men will easily recall and discuss early childhood memories of feeling different and bad, which they connect to their homosexuality. These recollections are important to explore, yet the skilled clinician must also lead his or her client in an exploration of experiencing difference that has its etiology before feelings for members of the same sex began to emerge (Shernoff and Finnegan, 1991). Once explored, this early sense of being different can relate to family secrets such as a parent's drinking, childhood sexual abuse, or simply to being the only one in the family not interested in sports.

Social workers should also understand that growing up gay in a heterosexual family is, by its very nature, a dysfunctional process unless the family is not homophobic (Shernoff and Finnegan, 1991). This is not to say that being gay is dysfunctional; rather, when people grow up in a family system where they cannot be or acknowledge who they truly are, they are placed in a system of dysfunction. A gay youth then must create a false self that he presents to his family in order to survive. Very often the gay adult is still maintaining a false self in some components of his life, whether it be work, family, or with nongay friends. The intrapsychic toll that this takes and how it is manifested in either symptoms of depression or anxiety are often the material of psychotherapeutic treatment with gay men. The toll of hiding one's true self must be identified and validated in order for the gay man to be able to move on and develop a positive gay image not based on shame and the need to hide (Shernoff and Finnegan, 1991).

Developmentally Disabled Gay Men

Mentally retarded gay men, like all others who are mentally handicapped, have sexual needs. If the retardation is not severe and the individual is able to live independently, then he is likely able to find partners as part of his adjustment to adulthood. Social workers in agencies that serve this population must take the lead in developing interventions that teach safer sexual practices regarding preventing AIDS.

Smith (1988) explains that for those with a severe handicap, the attitudes of caregivers are important. Expressing a need for sexual release may be viewed as "acting out," rather than the expression of a legitimate need, especially if the sexual desires are for a person of the same sex. On the other hand, professionals who condone or facilitate sexual expression between gay clients may find themselves vulnerable to accusations of "condoning" homosexuality, which in fact they are.

CHRONICALLY MENTALLY ILL GAY MEN

Gay men with severe psychopathology who have had multiple psychiatric hospitalizations are often clients in day treatment programs. Social workers in these settings need to be alert to gay clients, and how issues pertaining to their sexual orientation may exacerbate psychiatric symptoms. Ball (1994) discusses how these clients' psychosocial potential can be maximized in a group that addresses issues relating to their sexual orientation, including their double stigmatization as both mental patients and homosexuals. Ball also notes that psychiatrically disabled gay and lesbian clients must often leave their rehabilitation program to find support for their social and sexual needs. Yet in more mainstream settings within the gay community, these clients report feeling awkward because of their mental health history. Houston-Hamilton, Day, and Purnell, (1989) discuss that like all people, clients who are severely emotionally disturbed need education about AIDS that is customized for them.

SUBSTANCE ABUSE

Stall and Wiley (1988) reported that gay men not only used drugs more often but used a greater variety of drugs than did heterosexual men, and Shernoff (1983) reported incidence of injected drug use among middle-class, gay white men. Despite different geographic areas and sampling methods used in studies, there is strong evidence that gay men have more problems related to substance abuse than do heterosexuals (McKirnan and Peterson, 1989). Explanations for this phenomenon include internalization of society's homophobia, nonacceptance of self, fear of coming out, leading a double life, and low self-esteem (Finnegan and McNally, 1987; Kus, 1988, 1995; McKirnan and Peterson, 1989).

Faltz (1988) notes that often gay men have sought treatment for relationship difficulties, depression, anxiety, compulsive behavior, or phobias and have never been asked about, nor have they mentioned their drug or alcohol use. Thus, social workers should be skilled at diagnosing substance abuse problems, and need to take an alcohol and drug use history of each gay client seeking clinical services.

Finnegan and McNally (1987) described the stages of coming out as lesbian or gay and how these experiences affect chemically dependent behavior. Commonly, a client may be in one stage of denial about his chemical dependency and in another about being gay. To be effective, the worker must assess both stages of denial in order to formulate an effective treatment plan. Ratner (1993) cautions that the clinician should be wary of clients who enter treatment claiming to be comfortable with their sexual orientation and therefore insist that talking about lifestyles is unnecessary.

Shernoff and Finnegan (1991) suggest that a client's chemical dependency is not always the only justifiable focus early in treatment. There are times when people's concerns about their sexual orientation may demand attention if they are to get or stay clean and sober. For instance, counselors need to recognize that sometimes it is very important to validate clients' bitter or pained assertions that homophobia has seriously contributed to their use of chemicals.

A worker in a detox unit or other substance abuse facility may encounter an individual who does not identify as gay or bisexual and who has trouble maintaining his sobriety. This kind of client has repeatedly relapsed into active use of chemicals even when attending AA meetings and ostensibly working his program. In an attempt to help the client make sense of why he is unable to remain sober, it can be helpful to explore with this client the possibility that he might be struggling with feelings or fantasies related to being attracted to other men, even if he has never acted on these feelings.

The AIDS epidemic has contributed to the urgency of addressing gay men's chemical dependency. Stall (1988) has documented that a majority of men who fail to practice safer sex to prevent the transmission of HIV are under the influence of alcohol and/or drugs. Greene and Faltz (1991) discuss treatment strategies for gay men with a history of sobriety who relapse upon learning that they have been exposed to HIV or after an AIDS diagnosis.

DOMESTIC VIOLENCE

Social workers must be alert to instances where a gay client is either a victim or perpetrator of domestic violence (Renzetti and Miley, 1996). According to Walber (1988), no group within the gay community, regardless of race, class, ethnicity, age, ability, education, politics, religion, or lifestyle is exempt from domestic violence. Gay men can be battered or abused by a lover, ex-lover, roommate, or family member.

The worker may have difficulty identifying either a batterer/abuser or a survivor. Being abusive is not determined by a gay man's size, strength, or economic status. Gay men who batter or abuse can be friendly, physically unintimidating, sociable, and charming. Gay men who are battered or abused can be strong, capable, and dynamic (Walber, 1988). The issue in domestic violence, however, is control, and it is this unequal power relationship that distinguishes battering from fighting. Reports from both batterers and survivors are that abuse and violence most often occur when the abusive individual is under the influence of alcohol and/or drugs.

It is important for the clinician to remember that it usually is no easier for a gay man to leave an abusive or violent relationship than for any other abused spouse to do so. Battering relationships are rarely *only* violent or abusive. Love, caring, and remorse are often part of the cyclical pattern of abuse. This cycle can cause a survivor to feel confused and ambivalent about the nature of the relationship (Walber, 1988).

ANTIGAY VIOLENCE

Berrill (1992) reports that thousands of episodes—including defamation, harassment, intimidation, vandalism, assault, murder, and other abuse—have been reported to police departments and to local and national organizations (National Gay and Lesbian Task Force Policy Institute, 1992); while countless more incidents have gone unreported. Wertheimer (1992) notes that although lesbians and gay men are prone to a level of victimization that far exceeds that of the nongay population, existing crime victim service networks have largely failed to acknowledge gay victims of violent crime. He further contends that regardless of whether this failure has resulted from ignorance, neglect, or conscious hostility, its consequence is that gay people still frequently suffer the often devastating consequences of victimization in isolation and silence. As a result, the initial physical and psychological injuries that follow an assault are compounded. Wertheimer (1992) also asserts that most crime victim service providers remain unfamiliar with and insensitive to the needs of gay crime victims. Consequently, gay men who report crimes committed against them frequently must choose between hiding their sexual orientation from the service providers or disclosing it and risking ridicule and revictimization.

Social workers can offer invaluable assistance to gay victims of antigay violence in a number of concrete ways. A gay client will desperately be in need of an ally who can assist during the period immediately following an attack. A social worker should be prepared to advocate for the client with both the local police precinct and prosecutor's offices by accompanying the survivor to police stations and to interviews with prosecutors. This support helps ensure that officials treat the survivor with sensitivity and respect.

Gay victims of hate crimes need skilled professional assistance in working through their responses to the attack, turning the initial trauma into a potential growth experience (Garnets, Herek, and Levy, 1992). Helping the client transform his experience from that of a victim to one of a survivor is key. Garnets and colleagues suggest that the cognition, "Bad things happen because I'm gay," can be reformulated to "Bad things happen." They also discuss the need for mental health workers to help survivors of antigay sexual assault to separate the victimization from their experience of sexuality and intimacy.

AGING

Berger (1984) states that older gays and lesbians are most vulnerable to social, economic, and psychological forces and therefore are likely to come to the attention of social workers. Berger's research found that the social recluse did exist, but most older gay men studied function in networks of friends, lovers, and family as well as social civic and religious organizations within the gay community. The same study found that the majority of respondents were still sexually active, but not as frequently as in their youth. Social workers serving the elderly must learn about these networks and use them as available resources for older gay clients to meet other people.

Older gay people need the same services as all older people (Berger, 1984; Quam, 1997). Berger (1980) found that older gay men reported less depression and fewer psychosomatic symptoms than younger gay men. Older men in the midst of a transition to a newly acquired gay identity may seek counseling for help with this passage (Berger, 1984). Social workers may also be of assistance in responding to an older gay client's request for a gay visitor from the friendly visiting service. Social workers in nursing homes can be helpful to elderly gay clients by trying to facilitate that roommates be other gay residents if so desired, or providing counseling to the male couple when one member is placed in a nursing home. Clinicians may also be called upon to provide bereavement counseling for the surviving partner of a gay couple.

AIDS

In order to work effectively with today's gay men, social workers simply cannot underestimate the pervasive impact that more than a decade of HIV/AIDS has had on gay male communities as well on individual and collective psyches. "Understanding that trauma creates an unexpected and dramatic shift in feelings of safety and connection to others is vital to comprehending the intrapsychic and interpersonal issues of many people affected by HIV/AIDS in the gay community" (Mancoske and Lindhorst, 1995, p. 30). Rofes (1996, p. 26) notes that "many gay men throughout America are suffering a wide range of psychological responses that extend beyond bereavement and grief. Some may be at the stage of simple grief or multiple loss, but many others are experiencing severe depression, mood disorders, trauma, chronic trauma and post-traumatic stress disorder." Rofes goes on to explain that he is not attempting to pathologize gay men, but rather seeks to document the critical psychological reactions to AIDS of contemporary gay men. Almost all gay men have been directly affected by HIV/AIDS. Every time a gay man has sex, he is reminded of the potential lethalness of an unprotected act. Most gay men living in large urban centers have had at least one friend or lover become ill and die. It is not uncommon for some men to have experienced many friends and in some cases entire friendship networks predecease them.

For both the uninfected and men living with HIV/AIDS the result is a chronic state of grieving and what has been termed "bereavement overload," which manifests itself in symptoms that are identical to posttraumatic stress disorder. Since the traumas are chronic, however, there is little opportunity for resolution of the situation or reduction of the precipitating stressors. As Mancoske and Lindhorst (1995, p. 33) state, "People in the gay community are struggling to create new models and definitions of 'family.'" The advent of HIV/AIDS further complicates this struggle. The caregiving provided within families of choice is fatiguing. Exhaustion becomes a major factor for individuals with multiple friends/partners/family members who have become ill. Few supports have been developed to provide relief. These supports are particularly underdeveloped in rural areas and overwhelmed in urban areas most heavily impacted by the epidemic (Mancoske and Lindhorst, 1995, p. 33).

HIV-NEGATIVE MEN

The psychodynamics of the impact of AIDS on the uninfected has just recently begun to explored in work by Odets (1995) and Ball (1996). The uninfected are a population in dire need of psychosocial supports that both provide a place for them to express their feelings about the impact that having survived the epidemic so far has on them. In addition, the lifesaving work of helping ensure that these men remain uninfected is often best accomplished in psychotherapy or groups composed only of HIV-negative gay men. These men often present with symptoms that are similar to post-traumatic stress syndrome and often include survivor guilt. With increasing frequency there are reports that some HIV-negative gay men behave in ways that place themselves at risk for becoming infected. Often these men report having difficulties adjusting to their roles as survivors. Their emotional distress must not be minimized or neglected in counseling. Odets (1995) explains that in many cases HIV-negative gay and bisexual men have a psychological experience—a personal and social identity—that is more that of a sick or dying man than that of many HIV-positive men.

An important dynamic that clinicians must remain alert to when working within this population is "survivor guilt" (Moon, 1992).

Odets (1995) describes how the clinical presentation of these clients is unusual. He states that the impact of AIDS on the man's community and sense of self creates an exceptionally potent stressor. Treatment consists of addressing the consequent depressive and manic defenses, fear for one's health, hypochondriacal anxiety, and sexual dysfunction (Odets, 1995).

LIVING WITH HIV AND AIDS

For men who are themselves infected or are symptomatic with full-blown AIDS, there are understandable worries about who will take care of them now that most of their friends have died. Living with AIDS in the second decade of the epidemic is a vastly different experience than it was in the early years of this plague. Today 5 percent of gay men who have a documented exposure to HIV for at least ten years are still remaining asymptomatic (Cao et al., 1995). The National Institutes of Health have labeled people who have a documented exposure to HIV for ten or more years and who remain asymptomatic "nonprogressors." Nonprogressors live with constant dread of their health status changing, and all of the corresponding anxieties that this brings. They have also seen numerous friends and loved ones become ill and die. They are ever vigilant for any indication that their lives have begun to move onto the path that they have watched so many others travel. This often results in these men suffering from symptoms of an anxiety disorder. A systemic mental health approach that helps these men identify remaining sources of social support and utilizing these supports is critical in order to maximize their psychosocial functioning.

In addition to the nonprogressors, there are now long-term survivors of AIDS. In 1990, the Centers for Disease Control and Prevention defined long-term survivors as individuals who have been diagnosed with a major opportunistic infection for at least three years and are alive with a reasonably good quality of life (Moore et al, 1991). Some of these individuals may still be employed full time. "When viewing HIV as a chronic, life-threatening illness, a strengths perspective helps orient clients to the long haul of being HIV positive or of being a long-term survivor" (Mancoske and Lindhorst, 1995, p. 36). Interventions include supportive counseling to help individuals sustain their intimate relationships while letting them express all of the discomfort that accompanies living with such a stressful and uncertain condition.

Remien and Wagner (1995) find that mental health professionals can help clients manage the following issues: uncertainty about the future, grief reactions to multiple loss, accessing support networks, romantic relationships, managing a satisfactory relationship with primary care physicians, deciding about treatment options, the progression of symptoms, and career decisions. With many of these individuals, numerous therapeutic hours are spent evaluating the costs versus the benefits of going on full-time disability before they become too debilitated to enjoy retirement. Remien and Wagner (1995) specify that therapeutic tasks include validating emotional reactions, focusing on short-term goals, facilitating feelings of empowerment, obtaining concrete services, assessing psychiatric risk and suicidal ideation, promoting adaptive coping strategies, fostering family communication and cooperation, and talking about the meaning of death and dying.

HIV antibody testing centers, community-based AIDS service organizations (Lopez and Getzel, 1984), hospitals, home health care services, and private practice are all settings where gay men receive social work services. With the onset of AIDS, gay men seek therapy for a variety of new reasons: fears about getting AIDS (Forstein, 1984), the trauma of learning one is HIV positive, telling one's parents about a diagnosis of HIV seropositivity or of AIDS, learning to live with AIDS, exploring new priorities, approaching the end of one's life, and bereavement overload as a result of decimated friendship groups.

In addition to helping clients with AIDS obtain needed services and benefits, social workers have an important role to play in providing psychosocial support to those living with AIDS and their loved ones (Gambe and Getzel, 1989; Getzel, 1991; Lloyd and Kuszelewicz, 1995; Shernoff, 1990). A key component of psychotherapy with this population is to help clients manage the anxiety disorders that are probably the most frequent psychiatric complications of HIV disease in both those who are uninfected, yet at high risk, as well as those symptomatic of HIV disease (Dilley and Boccellari, 1989). Depression in people with AIDS and symptomatic HIV disease is common (Dilley and Boccellari, 1989); clinicians must be alert to the possibility that the depression can be organic in origin and usually responds well to psychotropic medication. Helping clients balance hope with the realities of living with a life-threatening illness is another essential component of counseling.

DEATH AND DYING

According to Dworkin and Kaufer (1995),

> The bereavement process experienced by gays and lesbians who experience losses due to HIV/AIDS must be understood as a chronic state of mourning. The implications of overlapping losses where the onset of mourning for one loss overlaps with the end stage of mourning for another loss are significant. Complicating this chronic state are post traumatic stress, loss saturation, unresolved grief, survivor guilt, and fear of infection with HIV. (p. 42)

Not only are gay men losing those with whom they have shared strong emotional ties, but they are also losing acquaintances, role models and co-workers at a very fast rate" (Dean, Hall, and Martin, 1988, p. 55). Thus, individual clinicians have to be prepared to assume a role of support and bearing witness that transcends traditional psychotherapy or counseling. The experience of many urban gay men is similar to that of a survivor of a catastrophe, and must be addressed with this understanding and within this context. Doka (1989) explains the concept of *disenfranchised grief,* which occurs when (a) the relationship is not recognized, (b) the loss is not recognized, and (c) the griever is not recognized. These are ordinary experiences for many gay men mourning a friend, lover, or community. As Dworkin and Kaufer (1995, p. 43) correctly note, "All of these factors must be taken into account in redefining the process of grieving and identifying the coping mechanisms and interventions appropriate for responding to the needs of today's gay men."

Following the death of his lover, the surviving partner may not receive condolences from family or workers who do not view a gay relationship as the equivalent of a marriage. This absence of understanding and support only increases the pain and anger surrounding his loss. Social workers doing individual counseling must be aware of these additional issues, which have an impact upon a gay man's grieving process, and find ways to elicit feelings of anger and shame that may surface in the absence of appropriate support while also actively consoling the grieving partner. Referring gay widowers to an AIDS bereavement group is often one helpful intervention in assisting the surviving partner to work through his grief.

Dworkin and Kaufer (1995) suggest that bereavement interventions also need to respond to developmental issues, existential themes, multiple and chronic primary and secondary losses, and the collective nature of grieving. They must be gay affirmative in addressing lowered self-esteem, personal identity, and questions about body image, and need to address the reestablishment of meaning in one's life. Many authors cited by Dworkin and Kaufer emphasize that social support is the key to coping with any loss, especially multiple loss. Yet with many entire friendship networks being wiped out by this plague, the therapist assumes a role and significance that may be a combination of counselor, friend, significant other, and just fellow human being. The weekly sessions may be the only remaining ongoing regular contact with any individual with whom the client has a history.

Talking About Dying

Any social worker in practice with gay men with AIDS has to be adept at knowing how and when to introduce topics about dying into the clinical conversations. As people develop symptoms of advanced AIDS they increasingly lose control over their bodies and lives. One task of counseling is to help people living with HIV and AIDS recognize what they can control. Clients living with HIV require help in planning for hospitalizations and debilitating illnesses. It is best to raise the difficult and painful issues associated with executing wills, advanced medical directives, living wills, and medical proxies long before there is any apparent need for them. One major issue for dying people is that they are at a point where their ability to control what happens to them has been greatly diminished. Clients at the end of their lives can be greatly empowered by therapists or counselors engaging them in a discussion about where they want to die. Many clients may not realize that whether to die at home, in the hospital, or in a hospice is a decision that they and their loved ones can and should consciously make together in consultation with the physician. It can be enormously helpful if the clinician or hospital social worker raises the issue of and explains the concept of hospice care.

It can often be difficult for all concerned to acknowledge that "enough is enough." It is an essential and completely appropriate role of the counselor to encourage the client to explore his or her feelings about whether or not to cease treatments or to continue fighting for extra time. It is not the worker's role to give permission for one choice or another. Dying can be a quality time both for the terminally ill person as well as those who love him. One way to help ensure this is for the worker to ask the client questions that will offer him or her options and some control over the process.

Crucial Questions to Ask a Dying Client

- Do you feel that you are going to die soon? If so, how do you feel about this?
- How will you know you no longer wish to continue medicines, treatments, or supplemental feedings? (It's important to reflect to the client that what he or she feels is intolerable may in fact change. Most people with AIDS surveyed felt that blindness, dementia, and incontinence were hallmark's of life not being worth continuing.)
  - Do you prefer to die at home, in a hospice, or in a hospital?
  - Whom do you wish to be with?
  - Would you like to have a clergy person make a final visit?
  - Is there anything you haven't said to your loved ones?
  - Is there anything else you need to do or complete?
  - Have you thought about letting go since it seems to me that you're suffering a great deal?

As Follansbee (1996, p. 6) states, "The dignity of a peaceful death, without pain, fear or futile therapy, can be realized only if time is spent in its preparation."

CONCLUSION

Individual clinical practice with gay men is suffused with the issue of illness, dying, surviving, and thriving as members of an oppressed population under siege by both a medical crisis as well as attacks by the Religious Right. State of the art interventions with this population in the 1990s needs to challenge traditional models of therapeutic intervention. While traditional psychotherapy is often still appropriate treatment, the skilled practitioner must be knowledgeable about and ready to employ a variety of case work, counseling, crisis intervention, and advocacy skills, in addition to intrapsychic exploration and a systems approach. By being eclectic in working with gay men, services are customized to meet diversified client needs. Gay men seeking clinical social work services often discuss issues that have the potential to bewilder and overwhelm the most skilled clinician. The work is intellectually demanding, often exhilarating, at times exhausting, and very rarely ever dull. The rewards for being flexible and creative in treatment approaches are tangible when clients invite and allow us to participate in their lives' journey. Contemporary practice with this population brings with it demands and challenges that reenforce the basic social work tenets of the need for regular, ongoing supervision, training, and supportive self-examination to help enable the practitioner to continue to make a skillful and disciplined use of his or her self in a sustainable fashion.

REFERENCES

American Psychiatric Association. (1987). *Diagnostic and Statistical Manual of Mental Disorders,* third edition (revised). Washington, DC: American Psychiatric Association.

Baez, E. (1996). Spirituality and the gay Latino client. In M. Shernoff (Ed.), *Human services for gay people: Clinical and community practice* (pp. 69-82). Binghamton, NY: Harrington Park Press.

Ball, S. (1994). A group model for gay and lesbian clients with chronic mental illness. *Social Work, 39*(1), 109-115.

Ball, S. (1996). HIV-negative gay men: Individual and community social service needs. In M. Shernoff (Ed.), *Human services for gay people: Clinical and community practice.* (pp.25-40). Binghamton, NY: Harrington Park Press.

Bayer, R. (1981). *Homosexuality and American psychiatry.* New York: Basic Books.

Berger, R. (1980). Psychological adaption of the older homosexual male. *Journal of Homosexuality, 5,* 161-175.

Berger, R. (1984). Realities of gay and lesbian aging. *Social Work, 29*(1), 57-62.

Berrill, K. (1992). Anti-gay violence and victimization in the United States: An overview. In G. Herek and K. Berrill (Eds.), *Hate Crimes,* (pp. 19-45). Newbury Park, CA: Sage Publications.

Bozett, R. (1981). Gay fathers: Evolution of the gay-father identity. *American Journal of Orthopsychiatry, 51*(3), 552-559.

Breeze. (1985). Social service needs and resources in rural communities. In H. Hidalgo, T. Peterson, and N. Woodman (Eds.), *Lesbian and gay issues: A resource manual for social workers* (pp. 43-48). Silver Spring, MD: National Association of Social Workers.

Cao, Y., Qin, L., Zhang, L., Safrit, J., and Ho, D. (January 26. 1995). Virologic and immunologic characterization of long term survivors of human immunodeficiency virus type 1 infection. *New England Journal of Medicine, 332*(4), 90-99.

Carballo-Dieguez, A. (1989). Hispanic culture, gay male culture, and AIDS: Counseling implications. *Journal of Counseling & Development, 68*(1), 26-30.

Cass, V. (1979). Homosexual identity formation: A theoretical model. *Journal of Homosexuality, 4* (3), 219-235.

Chan, C. (1989). Issues of identity development among Asian-American lesbians and gay men. *Journal of Counseling & Development, 68*(1), 16-20.

Coleman, E. (1988). Assessment of sexual orientation. In E. Coleman (Ed.), *Integrated identity for gay men and lesbians: Psychotherapeutic approaches for emotional well-being* (pp. 9-24). Binghamton, NY: Harrington Park Press.

Davison, G. (1982). Politics, ethics and therapy for homosexuality. In E. Paul, J. Weinrich, J. Gonsiorek, and M. Hotvedt (Eds.), *Homosexuality: Social, psychological and biological issues* (pp. 89-98). Beverly Hills, CA.: Sage.

Dean, L., Hall, W., and Martin, J. (1988). Chronic and intermittent AIDS-related bereavement in a panel of homosexual men in New York City. *Journal of Palliative Care, 4*(4), 54-57.

De la Vega, E. (1995). Considerations for presenting HIV/AIDS information to U.S. Latino populations. In W. Odets and M. Shernoff (Eds.), *The second decade of AIDS: A mental health practice handbook* (pp. 255-274). New York: Hatherleigh Press.

Dilley, J. and Boccellari, A. (1989). Neuropsychiatric complications of HIV infection. In J. Dilley, C. Pies, and M. Helquist (Eds.), *Face to face: A guide to AIDS counseling* (pp. 138-151), Berkeley, CA: Celestial Arts.

Doka, K. (1989). *Disenfranchised grief: Recognizing hidden sorrow.* Lexington, MA: Lexington Books.

Dworkin, J. and Kaufer, D. (1995). Social services and bereavement in the gay and lesbian community. In G. Lloyd and M. A. Kuszelewicz (Eds.), *HIV disease: Lesbians, gays and the social services* (pp. 41-60). Binghamton, NY: Harrington Park Press.

Faltz, B. (1988). Substance abuse and the lesbian and gay community: Assessment and Intervention. In M. Shernoff and W. Scott (Eds.), *The sourcebook on lesbian/gay health care,* second edition (pp. 151-161). Washington, DC: National Lesbian/Gay Health Foundation.

Finnegan, D. and McNally, E. (1987). *Dual identities.* Center City, MN: Hazelden.

Follansbee, S. (1996). The dying process. *FOCUS: A Guide to AIDS Research and Counseling, 11*(2), 5-6.

Forstein, M. (1984). AIDS anxiety in the "worried well." In S. Nichols and D. Ostrow (Eds), *Psychiatric implications of acquired immune deficiency syndrome* (pp. 49-60). Washington, DC: American Psychiatric Press.

Gambe, R. and Getzel, G. (1989). Group work with gay men with AIDS. *Social Casework, 70*(3), 172-179.

Garnets, L., Herek, G., and Levy, B. (1992). Violence and victimization of lesbians and gay men: Mental health consequences. In. G. Herek and K. Berrill (Eds.), *Hate crimes,* (pp. 207-226). Newbury Park: Sage.

Germain, C. B. (1978). General-systems theory and ego psychology: An ecological perspective. *Social Service Review,* 535-550.

Germain, C. B. (1980). Social context of clinical social work. *Social Work,* 483-488.

Germain, C. B. (1981). The ecological approach to people-environment transactions. *Social Casework,* 323-331.

Getzel, G. (1991). Survival modes for people with AIDS in groups. *Social Work 36,* (1), 7-11.

Gitterman, A. and Germain, C. B. (1976). Social work practice: A life model. *Social Service Review,* 601-610.

Gonsiorek, J. (1982). The use of diagnostic concepts in working with gay and lesbian populations. *Journal of Homosexuality, 7*(2/3), 9-20.

Gonsiorek, J. and Rudolph, J. (1991) Homosexual identity: Coming out and other developmental events. In J. Gonsiorek and J. Weinrich (Eds), *Homosexuality: Research implications for public policy* (pp. 161-176). Newbury Park: Sage.

Greene, D. and Faltz, B. (1991). Chemical dependency and relapse in gay men with HIV infection: Issues and treatment. In M. Shernoff (Ed.), *Counseling chemically dependent people with HIV illness* (pp. 79-90). Binghamton, NY: The Haworth Press.

Gunter, P. (1988). Rural gay men and lesbians in need of services and understanding. In M. Shernoff and W. Scott (Eds.), *The sourcebook on lesbian/gay health care,* second edition (pp. 49-53). Washington, DC: National Lesbian/Gay Health Foundation.

Herek, G. M. (1990). Homophobia. In W. R. Dynes (Ed.), *Encyclopedia of Homosexuality* (pp. 552-554). New York: Garland.

Houston-Hamilton, A., Day, N., and Purnell, P. (1989). Educating chronic psychiatric patients about AIDS. In J., Dilley, C. Pies, and M. Helquist (Eds.), *Face to face: A guide to AIDS counseling* (pp. 199-209). Berkeley: Celestial Arts.

Icard, L. (1985-86). Black gay men and conflicting social identities: Sexual orientation verses racial identity. *Journal of Social Work and Human Sexuality*, *4*(1-2), 83-93.

Isay, R. (1989). *Being homosexual: Gay men and their development*. New York: Avon Books.

Kinsey, A., Pomeroy, W. B., and Martin, C. E. (1948). *Sexual behavior in the human male*. Philadelphia: W. B. Saunders.

Kus, R. (1988). Alcoholism and non-acceptance of gay self: The critical link. *The Journal of Homosexuality, 15*(1/2), 25-41.

Kus, R. J. (Ed.). (1995) Addiction and recovery in gay and lesbian persons [Special Issue]. *Journal of Gay and Lesbian Social Services, 2*(1).

Lloyd, G. A. and Kuszelewicz, M.A. (Eds.). (1995). HIV disease: Lesbians, gays, and the social services. [Special Issue]. *Journal of gay and Lesbian Social Services, 2*(3/4).

Loiacano, D. (1989). Gay identity issues among black Americans: Racism, homophobia, and the need for validation. *Journal of Counseling & Development, 68*(1), 21-25.

Lopez, D. and Getzel, G. (1984). Helping gay AIDS patients in crisis. *Social Casework, 65*(7), 387-394.

Mancoske, R. and Lindhorst, T. (1995). The ecological context of HIV/AIDS counseling: Issues for lesbians and gays and their significant others. In G. Lloyd and M. A. Kuszelewicz (Eds.), *HIV disease: Lesbians, gays and the social services* (pp. 25-40). Binghamton, NY: Harrington Park Press.

Martin, A. (1984). The emperor's new clothes: Modern attempts to change sexual orientation. In E. Hetrick and T. Stein (Eds.), *Innovations in psychotherapy with homosexuals* (pp. 23-58). Washington, DC: American Psychiatric Press.

Martin, A. (1993). *The lesbian and gay parenting handbook*. New York: Harper-Collins.

McKirnan, D. and Peterson, P. (1989). Alcohol and drug use among homosexual men and women. *Addictive Behaviors, 14*, 545-553.

Moon, T. (1992). Survivor guilt in HIV negative gay men. Unpublished manuscript, San Francisco, CA.

Moore, R. D., Hidalgo, J., and Sugland, B. et al. (1991). Zidovudine and the natural history of the acquired immunodeficiency syndrome. *New England Journal of Medicine, 324*, 1412-1416.

Moses, A. and Bucker, J. (1980). The special problems of rural gay clients. *Human Services in the Rural Environment, 5*(5), 22-27.

National Gay and Lesbian Task Force Policy Institute. (1992). *Anti-gay/lesbian violence, victimization and defamation in 1991*. Washington, DC: National Lesbian/Gay Task Force.

Odets, W. (1995). *Life in the shadows: Being HIV negative in the age of AIDS*. New York: Irvington Press.

Quam, J. (Ed.) (1997). Social service for senior gay men and lesbians. [Special Issue]. *Journal of Gay and Lesbian Social Science, 6*(1).

Ratner, E. (1993). Treatment issues for chemically dependent lesbians and gay men. In L. Garnets and D. Kimmel (Eds.), *Psychological perspectives on lesbian and gay male experiences* (pp.567-578). New York: Columbia University Press.

Remien R. and Wagner G. (1995). Counseling long term survivors of HIV/AIDS. In W. Odets and M. Shernoff (Eds), *The second decade of AIDS: A mental health practice handbook* (pp. 179-200). New York: Hatherleigh Press.

Renzetti, C.M. and Miley, C.H. (Eds.). (1996). Violence in gay and lesbian domestic partnerships [Special Issue]. *Journal of Gay and lesbian Social Sciences, 4*(1).

Rofes, E. (1996). *Reviving the tribe: Regenerating gay men's sexuality and culture in the ongoing epidemic.* Binghamton, NY: Harrington Park Press.

Ross, M. (1983). *The married homosexual man: A psychological study.* London: Routledge and Kegan Paul.

Shernoff, M. (1983 Oct. 10-23). Nice boys and needles. *New York Native,* pp. 7-8.

Shernoff, M. (1984). Family therapy for lesbian and gay clients. *Social Work, 29*(4), 393-396.

Shernoff, M. (1990). Why every social worker should be challenged by AIDS. *Social Work, 35*(1), 5-8.

Shernoff, M. (1996). Gay men choosing to be fathers. In M. Shernoff (Ed.), *Human services for gay people: Clinical and community practice* (pp. 41-54). Binghamton, NY: Harrington Park Press.

Shernoff, M. and Finnegan, D. (1991). Family treatment with chemically dependent gay men and lesbians. *Journal of Chemical Dependency Treatment, 4*(1), 121-135.

Smith, J. (1988). Psychopathology, homosexuality and homophobia. In M. Ross (Ed.), *Psychopathology and psychotherapy in homosexuality* (pp. 59-74). Binghamton, NY: The Haworth Press.

Stall, R. (1988). The prevention of HIV infection associated with drug and alcohol use during sexual activity. In L. Siegel (Ed.), *AIDS and substance abuse,* (pp.73-80). Binghamton, NY: Harrington Park Press.

Stall, R. and Wiley, J. (1988) A comparison of alcohol and drug use patterns of homosexual and heterosexual men. *Drug and Alcohol Dependence, 22,* 63-73.

Sullivan, G. (Ed.). (1995). Gays and lesbians in Asia and the Pacific: Social and human services [Special Issue]. *Journal of Gay and Lesbian Social Services, 2*(2).

Tafoya, T. and Rowell, R. (1988). Counseling gay and lesbian native Americans. In M. Shernoff and W. Scott (Eds.), *The sourcebook on lesbian/gay health care,* second edition (pp. 63-67). Washington, DC: National Lesbian/Gay Health Foundation.

Theriot, K. (1993a, April), Reparative therapy [Letter to the editor]. *NASW News,* p.12.

Theriot, K. (1993b, October), "Reparative" response [Letter to the editor]. *NASW News,* p.14.

Walber, E. (1988). Behind closed doors: Battering and abuse in the lesbian and gay communities. In M. Shernoff and W. Scott (Eds.), *The sourcebook on lesbian/gay health care,* second edition (pp. 250-258). Washington, DC: National Lesbian/Gay Health Foundation.

Wertheimer, D. (1992). Treatment and service interventions for lesbian and gay male crime victims. In. G. Herek and K. Berrill (Eds.), *Hate Crimes* (pp.19-45). Newbury Park: Sage.

Wyers, N. (1987). Homosexuality in the family: Lesbian and gay spouses. *Social Work, 32*(2), 143-148.

Chapter 5

Individual Practice with Lesbians

Audrey I. Steinhorn

Homosexuality is assuredly no advantage, but it is nothing to be ashamed of, no vice, no degradation. It cannot be classified as an illness . . . Many highly respected individuals of ancient and modern times have been homosexuals, several of the greatest men among them (Plato, Michelangelo, Leonardo da Vinci, etc.). . . .

–Sigmund Freud
"Letter to an American Mother"

Female sexuality has a long history of being denied and, as evidenced by the above quote, lesbian sexuality has been denied even more specifically. In spite of this, today's lesbian community consists of as varied a group of women as one will find anywhere in Western society. Like most invisible minority groups, in this case a marginalized, stigmatized sexual one, they are frequently misunderstood. Lesbians do not have identifiable features such as color, age, or various specific physical attributes; but they do come in all shapes, ages, colors, and sizes, and with as many numerous stereotypes. One of the most common stereotypes assumes lesbians to be tough and masculine. This, however, is a stereotype that some lesbians and some heterosexual women both may fit.

Since most lesbians are not easily identifiable, it is important when working with women, that heterosexuality not be presumed or that prejudgments not be made about women who may fit some of these stereotypes.

WHO IS YOUR CLIENT?

When contemplating social work with lesbian clients, it is important to define what constitutes a lesbian. "Lesbian" is not a singular construct. The popular theory is that "lesbian" connotes sexual behavior. This is an erroneous assumption. The fact is that most women have more emotional social freedom to express feelings between themselves, which facilitates women's ways of relating to women. Many women who have strong emotional ties to women may identify as lesbian. There are women who have strong sexual involvements with some women or a particular woman who may not self-identify as a lesbian. Women who identify as lesbian may have feminist political beliefs yet relate to both men and women sexually or affectionately. Lesbianism, in this case, is more a way of life; not a sexuality issue. It is important to differentiate the above since the presence of one does not necessarily lead to the other. Currently, women who have sex with other women but do not identify as lesbian refer to themselves as "women who partner with women."

A further consideration is bisexuality. Many women, both single and married, establish emotional and physical relationships with people of both genders. Of these, some self-identify as bisexual, some as lesbian, and some as heterosexual. It is important not to assume anything about anyone until they have had a chance to self-identify. The use of unbiased language (i.e, do you have a significant other? Is that person a man or a woman?) can be helpful in finding out how a person self-identifies. It should also be noted that a client's self-identified sexual orientation may not reflect a stable or exclusive pattern. An identification of sexual orientation can also not be based on marital status or the presence or absence of children. Often lesbians are heterosexually married and many have children (McDonald and Steinhorn, 1993).

MARRIED LESBIANS

In Western society, heterosexuality and marriage are seen as synonymous. Being a lesbian is associated with being unmarried (Simon, 1987). Very little attention is given to the idea that many married and single women self-identify as lesbian or bisexual. One needs to be prepared to be open to all possibilities.

Lesbians have heterosexually married for a variety of reasons (Wyers, 1987). Leading a double life can and often does cause great stress for the married lesbian due to the pressures of multiple identities and the discontinuity of public and private life (Germain and Gitterman, 1996; Germain, 1981). This may be a source of guilt, shame, and self-hatred. Social workers need to be alert to their own tendencies of wanting to make things better and/or of wanting to change their client. They do not have "to do" anything but listen to their client and help her define her own needs and feelings as she determines the course of her life (e.g., What do you need to help you at this time? How can I be of help? What would you like to see happen in the near future? What changes would you like to make?). This is crucial because the belief that lesbianism and bisexuality are undesirable continues to prevent these women from acknowledging themselves and sharing this knowledge with friends and family. Internalized homophobia (the irrational fear and/or hatred of anyone or anything connected with homosexuality) is a debilitating negative force that drains self-esteem, makes one very fearful, and fosters a negative self-image.

One of the many varied roles of the social work practitioner is to understand that same-sex partner preference develops separate and apart from whatever other emotional processes are developing—including personality and characterological traits or disturbances. These traits and disturbances may affect or determine how a lesbian relates to others (i.e., affectionately, aggressively, dependently, sensitively); but they are independent of her sexual preference. A lesbian identity does not predict how a lesbian will behave.

This is not to suggest that lesbians do not encounter external problems that may lead to stressful conditions in their life, such as discrimination with housing, in child custody cases, and on the job (Germain and Gitterman, 1996; Germain, 1981). These experiences frequently evoke those special fears related to being different. Some adolescents and women can accept their identity with little turmoil while others may become fearful and confused by issues of isolation, stigma, and threats of/or actual violence, which can and does exert severely negative influences. These may lower self-esteem, heighten suspiciousness, and cause pervasive anxiety and/or debilitating sadness and depression.

Although therapeutic goals need to include helping the client deal with the affects of negative stereotypes and development of the recognition that difference does not mean that a person is inferior, professional responsibility does not end there.

As professionals, social workers also have an affirmative obligation to make society less hostile to lesbian and gay people.

ADOLESCENTS

Sexuality is usually not a topic with which adults are comfortable. This includes many social workers and therapists, who need to be aware of their reactions during discussions on the topic. Adolescents are frequently limited by societal expectations and assumptions of heterosexuality. Problems can arise for lesbian youth as they often have no one to talk to about their same-sex attractions; nor can they trust themselves to reveal their feelings to the people to whom they are attracted because of their fear of ridicule, rejection, and/or physical assault. Poor school performance, underdeveloped socialization skills, substance abuse, suicidal ideation or attempts, and running away from home are behaviors that have been seen in adolescents who are hiding their "secret" to avoid being labelled (DeCrescenzo, 1994; Schneider, 1989).

Despite significant increases in positive lesbian media visibility, it is still more usual that a girl who becomes aware that she is more attracted to girls than to boys will be secretive about this information. She may feel overwhelmed by confusion, fear, and anxiety, and wonder whether there is something wrong with her. She may also experience excitement as she explores a new sense of herself. However, just as she is discovering something very special about herself, she may find that she feels very much alone. She may not know who she can talk to, trust to keep her secret, and accept her even though she is "different."

This process of discovering an attraction and preference for members of the same sex is called "coming out." Coming out for a lesbian is a time to focus on ways she differs from the mainstream of the population. Cass (1979) has defined six stages in the process of coming out. Coming out is a lifelong process that all people experience when they allow themselves and/or others to discover who they really are (Grier and Cassidy, 1995). Coming out usually refers to those elements of the person that are the most difficult for her and others to accept. One of the most confusing aspects of the coming-out process is that of not knowing in advance when one is going to meet with a negative response. This may cause some to hide important information about themselves from others—a process that is referred to as "being in the closet."

GENDER BIAS

Lesbians tend to remain closeted more often than gay men not only because of their choice of life partner but also because of economic discrimination. Achieving job equality is hard enough for women without adding the additional burden of lesbianism. Gender bias is a burden for lesbians because language (use of primarily male pronouns) and institutions (entry-level jobs for women) all support and encourage a sub-par relationship to men. Gay males, even though they are discriminated against, are still male and enjoy the many privileges accorded their gender. This is important to bear in mind since there may be an assumption, because they both are homosexual, that lesbians and gay men have more in common than they do. This is not necessarily true. Many women's mental image of their own potential is still limited by gender bias and, for lesbians, compounded by homophobia.

Women are often the target of physical violence, and, consequently, lesbians are often at risk for being the target of violent hate crimes (Berrill, 1992). In recent years, there has been more public reporting of the violence against lesbians, which has not been limited to assault or rape but also includes murder.

One might wonder why anyone would choose to be a lesbian if there is so much antigay violence everywhere. Most lesbians do not choose their sexual orientation just as most heterosexual people do not choose theirs. More lesbians are choosing not to deny who they are and are coming out to themselves and to others despite the fact that it makes them vulnerable to harassment and possible physical harm (Berrill, 1992; Garnets, Herek, and Levy, 1992).

COUPLES

Multiple identity issues exist for lesbians in couples as well as for individual lesbians. Juggling these multiples can cause considerable stress and discontinuity in a woman's life because of role expectations that not only conflict with each other but are ultimately incompatible. An example of this is a woman who is not out to her family, acts like a heterosexual daughter, is perceived as heterosexual, and is actually in a lesbian relationship that is not acknowledged by anyone including herself. This limits her ability to participate fully as a partner and continues her image as single.

Variations on the above scenario include being single at work and in other settings while being in a couple and socializing primarily with lesbians in ones private life; and identifying as "friends" instead of as a couple and calling one's partner a roommate. How many heterosexual women are known to not acknowledge their conjugal partner? Not many. However, quite a few lesbians do not make this acknowledgement about their partners with the result that their relationship remains invisible, thus continuing the myth that lesbians do not have stable, long-term relationships.

Lesbian couples are similar to heterosexual couples in that they enter into a relationship for love, intimacy, companionship, economic support, and the opportunity to have, create, and raise a family. This may also, but not necessarily, include the idea of a relationship being committed, usually monogamous, and long term (Kurdek, 1994).

Keeping a relationship private or secret can cause many unforeseen problems that can affect its very stability. Ethnicity, age, class, religion, occupation, and previous sexual relationship history can affect how partners relate to each other in terms of individual lesbian identity development. The women may also be in different stages of lesbian identity development or have different expectations or experiences of being "out" in varying situations (Lewis, 1979). The presence of children, whether they represent a blended family or those born to the couple, can be a very significant dimension for a couple (Clunis and Green, 1993).

In addition to all of the above, it is important for the counselor working with lesbian couples (See Barranti and McVinney in this collection) to remember that the lack of legal protections and the absence of religious, social, and economic supports and sanctions affect them significantly. The homophobia of friends, family members, employers, co-workers, and neighbors and the threats of/or incidents of actual violence towards lesbians also need to be considered in deciding and implementing treatment goals with them that can realistically meet their needs (Berzon, 1988).

DOMESTIC VIOLENCE

Social workers dealing with couples need to be alert to a specific invisible problem of this often invisible minority. In Western society, dominance of one person over another is highly valued (Berzon, 1988; Renzetti and Miley, 1996). In addition to the usual conflict resolution problems that may need to be addressed, issues of power and control may need to be explored if the couple has difficulty with openness, vulnerability, equality, and cooperation.

Abusive relationships exist in the lesbian world although people rarely speak about them. Intimidation, emotional abuse, and physical violence occur just as they do in heterosexual relationships. In her study of lesbian battering, Hart (1986) distinguishes between violence and battering. The critical ingredient in her definition of battering is that the batterer uses violence or abusive behavior to gain power and control over her partner.

Social work counselors need to explore for possible abuse (e.g., Does your partner ever hurt you emotionally or physically? How? How often?). Women who know or think they are being abused need to get help (e.g., Have you called and gotten any assistance yet from a violence support group? Would you like my help in finding one?) Readings by Lobel (1986) and NiCarthy (1982, 1987) are recommended resources on the topic.

Some believe that it is not possible for women to do serious physical harm to others; this, however, is not true. Abuse and battering experiences in lesbian relationships are often sufficiently severe to cause symptoms of post-traumatic stress disorder (Hammond, 1989) such as social withdrawal, sleep disturbance, guilt, and dissociative incidents. One must be careful not to assign these symptoms to other diagnoses.

LESBIAN MOTHERS, CHILDREN, AND FAMILIES

Traditionally, lesbian mothers have been those who were un-aware of their lesbianism at the time of their marriage and the birth of their children or those who were aware but made a choice to marry and bear children instead of practicing an "unacceptable" lifestyle as a lesbian and dealing with the special fears of being different. Later in life, they made the choice to divorce and raise their children alone or with a lesbian partner. There will always be women who come out after marriage and divorce, and their children are usually accepted by others in their mothers' new community (Steinhorn, 1982).

For at least the last decade, more lesbians have been choosing to have children (Pies, 1985). They are doing it in a variety of ways: some use alternative donor insemination; some have a "planned pregnancy" through intercourse with a known and carefully selected donor; others adopt, either in this country or abroad. They do this either as a single parent or with a nonbiological coparent. Some lesbians may make an agreement with a gay male who wishes to father a child/family and also have a lesbian partner. The three may share child-rearing responsibilities. Many more variations of lesbian families exist (Hall, 1978; Schulenberg, 1985) and all have the po-tential to give a child a sense of love, family, and security. When children experience love and support from parents and sympathetic adults, they can usually deal with and master the stresses of growing up—even when they include being a member of an alternative family (Green, 1978; Kirkpatrick, Smith, and Roy 1981; Rafkin, 1990).

This process is not without problems. Insemination by friends may lead to custody problems. Nonbiological lesbian comothers rarely have rights by law and frequently lose contact with their child if the relationship with its biological mother ends. In addition, they often experience insensitivity on the part of schools and other insti-tutions to their family construct. Alternative donor insemination raises the thorny issue of rights: a child's right to know its origins/heritage; the mother's right to keep the truth of conception from her child; and the process of telling a child about its origins.

Formerly married lesbian mothers may experience visitation and custody problems, coming out issues, isolation and/or economic hardships (McDonald and Steinhorn, 1993). Lesbian parents are pioneers in many ways. They are both different from and similar to heterosexual parents. As such, they have to cope with many new, painful, lonely, exciting, happy feelings and experiences. They are in the unique position to learn from both groups if they can be supported to recognize, reach out for, and accept help (i.e., You could say, "Balancing all of these new experiences must be hard for you. How do you cope with your stress?").

LESBIANS OF COLOR

Just as all of us have some racist tendencies regardless of our skin color, everyone has some homophobia regardless of one's sexual orientation. As a white, middle-class lesbian, I approach the issue of racism with concern and I need to also be aware of my racism. I do not know what it feels like to be a member of a cultural or racial minority such as an African American (Cochron and Mays, 1988), Asian (Chan, 1989), or a Native American (Allen, 1984; Tafoya and Rowell, 1988) might. However, in addition to my minority member-ship as a woman and a lesbian, I have also experienced anti-Semitism and rejection by my family of origin and the dominant American culture. This can be very demoralizing and evocative of thoughts such as, "What do I have to do to prove that I'm OK?" Lesbians, especially lesbians of color, may need help to become aware of and learn how to deal with the particular stressors of com-ing out, homophobia (including their own), and their multiple identi-ties. In doing this, it is very important that social work practitioners help them understand that certain stressors are universal—not neces-sarily about them in particular—even if it feels like that. Helping clients learn to differentiate is an important therapeutic goal.

Working with lesbians of color and from diverse cultures calls upon professionals to deal with multiple cultural differences (See Hidalgo, 1995, and Walters in this collection). Additionally, practi-tioners need to reflect on their own biases. This is important espe-cially in view of the fact that Western society predominately reflects mainstream culture's heterocentric and racist values. Dispelling biases involves the acquisition of varied and specific cultural knowledge: the culture's attitude toward homosexuality and lesbianism, the role of nuclear and extended family in the culture, gender role expectations for women, the role of education for women, and the socioeconomic expectations for women. In addition, it is important for social workers to be aware of their assumptions and generalizations about individual cultures. Each cultural group has its unique differences. Generalizations from one culture to another would be counterproductive.

The social work practitioner must also take steps to be conscious not only of his or her own but also of his or her client's assumptions and generalizations about various cultures. For example, if the practitioner is white and the client is African American, the practitioner might want to say something like, "You never mentioned anything about the differences that exist between us. I wonder what it is like for you, a woman of color, to be working with me, a white woman/man?"

Another important factor is the client's primary identification. Is it to an ethnic (African American, Asian, Latina, Native American) group, or to their sexual orientation, or both? Cochron and Mays (1988) noted that African-American lesbians may be more likely to remain part of a heterosexual community for several reasons, including gender roles, the role of family, and ethnic and financial support. This identification is important for social workers to recognize and accept . Without it, clients will lack trust and may feel that their social workers have agendas of their own. Self-acceptance can free the client to deal with and be more open about the problems she is experiencing about being a lesbian.

Working with a Latina client may mean that in addition to looking for homophobia in her counselor's response to her, she also may be looking for the classism, racism, and colonialism that many Spanish-speaking people experience. In New York, many Latinas do not even speak Spanish. It is also crucial to be sensitive to gender roles—especially those relating to passivity, submissiveness, and the enhancement of the life and home of the primary male she is expected to have in her life. Since operating outside of the masculine-oriented society is not acceptable, Latina lesbians often conflict with their cultural ways of behaving and can experience significant identity issues, i.e., feeling like a displaced person (Bonilla and Porter, 1990). Here, the use of direct questions may be helpful: "I find that I may not have sufficient understanding of your family experience because I do not know enough about your culture. Can you tell me more about what it is like for you?"

DIFFERENTLY ABLED LESBIANS

Some impairments are visible and some are not. The degree of disability depends on the degree of impairment in one's functioning. In a highly physical and mobile society, those who cannot participate fully are often viewed and grouped into one undifferentiated and condescending category, "the disabled."

Unfortunately, it is often assumed that people with disabilities have no sexual feelings, whatever their sexual orientation. Many people with disabling conditions, including lesbians, have internalized these assumptions and do not believe in their ability to be sexual in different ways. Lesbians with disabling conditions need to be recognized as individuals with sexual desires and needs. Practitioners must be prepared not only to acknowledge this, but also to teach the techniques that will help them achieve sexual satisfaction.

Clearly this educational process is further complicated for lesbians since they are often isolated not only from other lesbians and gay men but also from other differently abled lesbians and gay men. Attitudes are not the only factors causing this isolation. Isolation can also be caused by the lack of physical accessibility. Poorly funded lesbian groups can often not afford accessible meeting space where differently abled lesbians can have the opportunity for social interaction and networking.

Often a differently abled lesbian goes through a process of denial, anger, depression, and resolution (Rubin, 1981) particularly related to loss. It is important to listen for signs of these feelings in order to be of utmost help to this group who have been mistreated, oppressed, and repressed. The inferior status awarded differently abled lesbians can engender rage that may not show but needs to be dealt with.

RURAL LESBIANS

While it may be true that more lesbians are coming out, that does not or may not mean that they are from rural areas where there tends to be a strong value placed on being heterosexual. With limited privacy, living in a small town is like living in a goldfish bowl. Rural living tends to be conservative. There is often a strong emphasis on "traditional" values, morals, and behavior. Women are expected to marry, raise a family, and be part of extended families and active members of church congregations.

Sameness is highly valued in Western society, which conditions individuals to be negatively biased toward people who are not perceived to be heterosexual. Typically, any woman who chooses not to marry is assumed to be either an old maid or a lesbian. Old maids are accepted, although looked upon with pity. It is easier to think of a single woman as an old maid than it is to think of her as being a lesbian (Simon, 1987). Lesbianism implies sexuality. Women are not expected to be sexual unless they are married. Lesbians are scorned because of their sexual preference in partners and they are very often rejected for being different. The pressure to follow the cultural norms is especially powerful in rural areas where it is much more difficult to be invisible than it is in urban areas. Heterosexual expectations can put significant stress on any woman's coping mechanisms and sense of well-being regardless of whether she is a lesbian or a heterosexual. However, if one is keeping her lesbianism a secret, the combination can cause heightened suspiciousness, anxiety, self-hatred, or depression as well as isolation. Many lesbians, especially those in rural areas, need help in learning how to deal with these stressors. They especially need help in learning how to differentiate when it is appropriate for them to stay in the closet (which it very often is) and when it is safe to self-disclose or come out of the closet. Asking questions such as "Where do you feel safest?" or "What are your fears?" might help to produce valuable understanding. This may be especially true for heterosexual social workers who have never been stigmatized or persecuted for their sexual orientation.

Confidentiality, the safeguarding of private information, is one of the cornerstones of the social work profession. Confidentiality is critical in working with lesbians in order to avoid "outing" them. Any inadvertent or purposeful statement or act that is likely to establish that a woman is lesbian or bisexual can be damaging. Since privacy, confidentiality, and/or anonymity are hard to maintain in rural areas, it is understandable that lesbians fear self-disclosure on most levels and that they may be extremely sensitive to having a sense of not being taken seriously about this, to not feeling understood, to not having their fears fully appreciated. The fear of being inadvertently outed is often so great for lesbians in rural areas that they may choose to travel many miles away from their hometowns to seek out therapy.

As is evident from the above, isolation can be a problem for all lesbians—especially those in rural areas where there are so few resources available. Health problems could also be an issue because of a lack of appropriate educational and health services specifically for lesbians. To help deal with social isolation, many lesbians travel great distances to be with other lesbians. Monthly potluck suppers are a popular means of networking. Here, lesbians from all around are able to get together in a safe setting, talk to others similar to them, and share personal experiences.

In working with rural lesbians, it is very important for the social worker to become as familiar as possible with the local culture and the nearest available resources. This will help the worker be more realistic about what is and is not possible in the client's community (Breeze, 1985; Gunter, 1988).

The following case vignette illustrates some of the relevance of the dimensions of rural lesbians and lesbians who are differently abled.

CASE VIGNETTE

Donna is a thirty-five-year-old bank teller who became paralyzed from the waist down as the result of a skiing accident. She lives in a small town approximately seventy miles out of Cleveland. Donna recently moved back to her own apartment, which was in the process of being modified for her use. Doors needed to be widened and bars placed in the bathroom.

After leaving the hospital, Donna had gone to a rehabilitation center for physical therapy and the acquisition of new skills. Donna was frightened to be going home on her own. She wasn't sure that she could manage by herself. A few of her friends had volunteered to "help" her but she wasn't sure what kind of help she needed. Donna wished that her ex-lover was around. Laura had had a great deal of trouble accepting Donna with her new disability and they had terminated their relationship. Donna was very angry and hurt by this. She was also concerned about ever getting a new lover. "After all, who could love a cripple?" she wondered. Donna was having significant difficulty accepting her changed body. Since she didn't accept it, she couldn't imagine how anyone else could.

Donna's social worker at the rehab center had led a group for people, which she found very helpful but also frustrating. Since everyone in the group was heterosexually identified, Donna did not talk about the loss of her partner. Fears of rejection plagued her because of her sexual orientation. Donna felt isolated and, at times, overwhelmed by sadness. Having no one to talk with about these feelings, Donna was becoming depressed and hopeless. She wanted to join a gay disabled group but didn't know where to begin to look for one nor how she would get to a meeting even if she found one.

Prior to her accident, Donna and Laura, who lived together as roommates, traveled to Cleveland to participate in lesbian social events and a potluck circle. Donna feared that she might never get there again since it would probably be a long time before she would be able to afford the necessary modifications for her car. Donna was not out to her family and she hardly felt able to ask them for help with transportation.

Social work practitioners may find that it is important to do more outreach than they are used to doing when they are working with clients like Donna. Home visits, telephone interviews, and e-mail may help to provide more ongoing and all important contact for people who are so often isolated. If you as a social worker suspect that your client may relate primarily to women, it will be important to explore your hunch or your idea with the use of unbiased language. If your idea is accurate, it is important to proceed slowly with your assessment. Any treatment planning should include realistic goals which your client considers to be feasible and which do not compromise her identity and/or anonymity. Pooling your client's knowledge of gay and lesbian resources can often lead to creative problem solving. Additional researching of gay and lesbian resources on the part of the practitioner can be a helpful supplement to your client's knowledge.

Most important, some of Donna's problems will occur because many of her issues are universal to all people and some will occur because she is not heterosexual. All of Donna's problems need equal professional attention.

HEALTH

All health care providers need to know the unique stressors in a lesbian's life in order to effectively deal with her medical issues. They need to understand that homophobia—the fear of and hatred toward lesbians, bisexuals, and gay men—causes many lesbians and bisexuals to avoid health care rather than face further negative reactions such as condescension, moralizing, neglect, intimidation, breach of confidentiality, and denial of care from the helping professionals (Peterson, 1996).

As a result of the above, many lesbian clients may not receive adequate or fundamental health care. The American system of health care is a very heterocentric system. There are very few systems like the Lesbian Health Program of the Community Health Project in New York City presently in existence. As a result, lesbians often do not have access to adequate health care education that could affect how they care for themselves. This is particularly important as lesbians often assume that they will not be affected by the same medical conditions as heterosexual women and they may not know what to ask for, what kind of medical assistance they may need, or where to go for proper medical assistance.

Many may not seek the medical care they feel they need because they lack the finances necessary for health insurance and/or doctors fees or may not be covered by a partner's insurance plan. In addition, if a lesbian does not have a primary physician, she may be reluctant to go to a family planning center or obstetric clinic—the traditional sources of preventive health care services for middle- and low-income women, whether single or married, lesbian or heterosexual.

This is unfortunate as lesbians need to have regular physical and gynecological exams just like heterosexual women. O'Hanlan (1995) suggests that lesbians are more likely to be overweight, have fewer children, and get less breast screening. Breast cancer, which affects many women, may be even more common among lesbians.

Lesbians, like all women, experience menopause. Although it is a natural event related to the diminishing supply of estrogen and the cessation of menstruation, it can involve a range of simple or complex changes. Good medical care can minimize complications. In some cases, women develop related emotional conditions that need to be addressed. These may include mood disorders and/or depression. Some symptoms may respond to relaxation techniques, visualization, and meditation, while others may respond to conventional therapeutic work.

Lesbians get sexually transmitted diseases (STDs) just as heterosexual women do. Lesbians get STDs from sex with other women regardless of their sexual experience with men. However, some women with whom they do have sex might have had sex with men, which then puts them at risk. The inaccurate assumption/belief that lesbians cannot get AIDS can be dangerous to the health and well-being of unsuspecting lesbians. Diseases that often occur are herpes, chlamydia, cystitis, pelvic inflammatory disease, warts, and vaginitis. These diseases need to be treated in lesbians just as they are with heterosexual women. If they go untreated, serious complications might develop. Bradford and Ryan (1988) found in their lesbian health care survey that many lesbians reported receiving no care for gynecological problems. The hesitancy that many lesbians have in seeking medical help on a regular basis is especially dangerous since many infections are asymptomatic. Also, HIV/AIDS in women frequently initially appears in the reproductive organs (Johnson, Smith, and Guether, 1987).

HIV/AIDS

During the initial phases of the AIDs pandemic, it was widely believed that lesbians were at a low risk for the AIDS virus not only because they were believed to have less sex with men but also because cases of AIDS among lesbians were not being counted or publicized (See Lloyd and Kuszelewicz, 1995). This was due to the way data was reported (Chu, Bushlee, Fleming, and Berkelman, 1990). This reporting was inaccurate primarily because it is not how a woman identifies that puts her at risk, it is her specific behavior. HIV-positive lesbians did then and do now exist, even though it wasn't until April 1995 that the Centers for Disease Control and Prevention called the first meeting to address woman-to-woman HIV transmission (Hansen, 1995).

Who is at risk? For the purpose of this chapter, self-identified lesbians who have sex with men or who use intervenous drugs are at greater risk than those who only have sex with women. Identifying as a lesbian does not mean that a female sexual partner has not been exposed to the virus. She could have been with a woman who had been with a man who had been exposed to the AIDS virus or used intravenous drugs. In addition, AIDS and other sexual diseases can be transmitted by artificial insemination from a donor who has not been properly screened.

Since current research has not produced sufficient information that is needed about women who have sex with women, social workers have to be sensitive to lesbian community issues including, but not limited to, sexuality and the discussion of sexuality; the social status of drug usage for lesbians and bisexuals; the relationship of drug use and sexual behavior; the homophobia in drug treatment and HIV/AIDS outreach programs; and the various subcultures a client may belong to (Division of HIV/AIDS Prevention, 1996).

Social workers need to educate themselves very specifically on issues of HIV/AIDS transmission, prevention, symptoms, and treatment for all women—and especially lesbians—because lesbians need to be taught to participate in safer sex practices, something they may not have been doing since they thought they could not get AIDS.

In addition to the above, social workers need to understand how the impact of HIV/AIDS on the gay male community affects the lesbian community. Many lesbians have gay friends, as do many couples who socialize with both men and women. Often when these men become HIV positive and/or develop AIDS, lesbians become part of the caregiving team. In the absence of a family of origin, lesbians often become primary care providers. Chronic emotional stress may develop from prolonged involvement, especially if the experience involves helping a person through the dying process (See Shernoff's paper in this text). In addition, some of these men may also have provided sperm for artificial insemination and/or helped to raise a lesbian's child/children. Loss then becomes an issue for the whole lesbian family. If the family does not have an aware and supportive circle of friends and extended family, they may go through the grieving process alone, become emotionally and physically depleted, and develop a complicated mourning process that will need to be explored and addressed in therapy (Dworkin and Kaufer, 1995).

A final note on health issues to keep in mind is that lesbian couples may face specific discrimination in medical and/or hospital settings. Partners are frequently excluded completely from medical participation because they are not "family," and hospitals often have visitation policies geared toward heterosexual marital or family of origin relationships. Insensitivity to lesbian and lesbian couple issues in drug treatment programs and HIV/AIDS outreach and inpatient programs aimed primarily toward men may prevent lesbians from disclosing their relationship or identity. If a couple is not public about their ties to each other, it would not occur to or be possible for them to draw attention to their relationship. This is especially true for older lesbians who often have internalized many generations of past homophobia. All lesbians dealing with this discrimination will need help to draw up powers of attorney, wills, personal living wills, and hospital living wills. A joint checking account, if one doesn't already exist, may also be helpful.

ALCOHOL AND SUBSTANCE ABUSE

In the March 1989 issue of *Our Voice,* published by the Pride Institute of Minneapolis, Minnesota, statistics were quoted that indicated that 33 percent of the gay and lesbian population is chemically dependent versus 10 to 12 percent of the general population having drug or alcohol problems (Deniston, 1989). These findings were consistent with an earlier study by Bradford and Ryan (1988). More recent data regarding lesbian alcohol abuse indicates rates no higher than those of heterosexual women surveyed in the Chicago and the San Francisco areas (Bloomfield, 1993; McKirnan and Peterson, 1989).

Both studies may be accurate for the populations they researched. Clubs or bars have been a place where lesbians and gay men have felt less fear of discrimination and more opportunity to socialize, network, and get information on events in the community (Kus, 1995). Earlier samples may have included more lesbians who went to bars—who tended to drink more. Later studies may not have reached sufficient women who did not frequent bars. Many lesbians do not go to bars, they just "drink at home," and some of these may drink more than lesbians who do go to bars. This is especially true for those in isolated social and geographical situations and those with addictive personalities. A final note: it is difficult to establish rates of prevalence in a largely hidden population.

Statistics aside, it is important to understand that there are pressures in Western society that encourage and support the use and abuse of various substances. Substance abuse is accepted and practiced by a large percentage of the U.S. population as there is a tradition of self-medicatation to avoid discomfort and pain. Within the lesbian community, alcohol and drugs have been such a significant part of the social scene that their use is taken for granted, not considered unusual or, more important, often thought not to be potentially harmful.

In addition to understanding the above, it is helpful to know what drugs people use and why (DeStefano, 1986). Social work practitioners must avoid the trap of using one's sexual orientation as a causative factor in substance abuse. As professionals, practitioners need to be sensitive to the fact that we may encounter situations in which we could inadvertently become enablers and help condone continued use or abuse (i.e., "I guess I'd drink too if I had all your problems").

Being different in mainstream society is difficult, but not everyone who is different drinks alcohol. Homophobia may be a very key factor in a lesbian's substance abuse problem. When the use of alcohol and other substances is rationalized away by the difficulties of life, which may or may not include homophobia, lesbians do themselves a disservice. The comment, "Who wouldn't want to get away from the pressures?" is just a part of denial that is very harmful to people with addictive behavior. It is clear that working through the acquisition of a lesbian identity requires a clear head. This includes being substance free.

For those who do want to do something about their problem, twelve-step programs can be helpful. In large cities, there are often many lesbian-only meetings available. In suburban or rural areas where the issue of disclosure may be more problematic, weekend trips to a city may be a solution. The combination of twelve-step programs and individual and group therapy is often very helpful, especially since there may be underlying depression present that would need to be addressed whatever its origin. Knowledge of substance use and/or need for abstinence is especially necessary if the use of antidepressants are therapeutically indicated (Johnson, Smith, and Guether, 1987).

OLDER LESBIANS

Growing older brings challenges, joys, problems, and hopefully wisdom (Kehoe, 1989; Quam, 1997). Age is relative—some people are old at 60, others at 80. Contrary to some beliefs that lesbians and gay men lead depressed, lonely lives, many have the exact opposite kind of life. They usually have developed support networks that they consider to be "family." Many older lesbians are so accustomed to living with stigma that being old is not necessarily as stigmatizing for them as it is for heterosexuals (Dorfman et al., 1995). They are more used to being self-reliant, have learned to support themselves financially, to plan for their future and anticipate for their financial lives when they are old.

Many older lesbians have developed a way of interacting that is unique to their generation and invisible to most other people (Deevy, 1990). While this way of presenting themselves to the outside world may have been an important way to protect them when they were younger, invisibility can work against them in their later years. When an older couple is not out, a problem can develop if one member of the couple is ill or dies. Her partner may not be able to go to the hospital, make medical decisions, or have the power to make sure that her rights will be protected in terms of joint property. Problems may also arise involving retirement homes or nursing homes. Policies may not permit same sex couples to purchase a home or, in the case of a nursing home, to share the same room. Older lesbians can, at times, need social work help with certain medical needs, bereavement counseling (Martin, 1991), and legal counseling. Often, if an individual or couple is out in the community, assistance can be arranged with a lesbian and/or gay resource center. Older lesbians have earned respect for their heritage and their history.

RELIGION

Everyone is reared with a sense of ethics, values, and morality learned from parental figures, religious institutions, schools, communities, and society at large. Parents teach children standards of conduct and moral judgments about behaviors, assisting children in learning "right" from "wrong." Such moral judgments may have significant meaning to lesbian, gay, and bisexual clients (Nelson, 1985).

The references about male homosexuality in the Bible, although erroneously interpreted, are well known and often quoted. According to Lovinger (1994), female homosexuality is never mentioned in the Old Testament, while New Testament references are vague. Despite this, self-esteem and self-worth of many lesbians have been adversely affected by many negative teachings of organized religion (Spong, 1992, 1994).

Clients can be done a disservice if practitioners do not address their spiritual and religious beliefs. Many people have been brought up with some kind of religious training. Whether it is a significant part of everyday life or not, it often becomes an integral part of life that has been deeply ingrained. Guilt and shame, both of which are often religiously driven, exert powerful influences. Addressing these feelings in work with clients can help them to be less judgmental of themselves and others and be more curious about their various reactions rather than just having them and reacting. As this process takes place, they will have the opportunity to learn that life is more complex than they had thought—that they can think about their reactions, try to understand them, and then decide how they wish to react. This new awareness can provide them with more options, a new sense of freedom, and a new sense of power in their lives.

CONCLUSION

It is said that maturity of mind is the capacity to endure uncertainty—a feeling that is universal to us all. Uncertainty is definitely a part of the lesbian and bisexual experience, and comes with the territory. It may also be an issue for the social work practitioner working with a lesbian or bisexual client. This may especially be true if the worker is unfamiliar with or has little experience with lesbians. This does not have to immobilize or overwhelm a worker. During the psychosocial assessment, knowledge of a client's strengths, abilities, and weaknesses can be acquired. Working with this knowledge can enhance the lesbian's ability to deal with uncertainty and strengthen her. Social workers need to understand that while uncertainty can add to personal stress, the lesbian's increased ability to deal with herself and her surroundings can become a special quality and personal asset for her.

Working with lesbian clients can be difficult and rewarding. As a values-based profession, social workers are challenged by the NASW Code of Ethics to recognize, accept, and value differences. How a lesbian deals with her differences and the problems they may bring is uniquely hers. There is no right way to deal with uncertainty. How she deals with it does not have to be radical but it must be personal. A major key to a full and productive life is how persons adapt to life and what life deals them (Germain, 1981; Germain and Gitterman, 1996). Practicing with clients from an informed and thoughtful perspective, professionals engaging lesbian clients can encourage clients to have fuller, happier, and more productive lives.

REFERENCES

Allen, P. (1984) Beloved women: The lesbian in American Indian culture. In T. Darty and S. Potter (Eds.) *Women Identified Women* (p. 96). Palo Alto, CA: Mayfield.

Berrill, K. (1992). Anti-gay violence and victimization in the United States: An overview. In G. Herek and K. Berrill (Eds.), *Hate Crimes* (pp. 19-45.) Newbury Park, CA: Sage.

Berzon, B. (1988). *Permanent partners: Building gay and lesbian relationships that last.* New York: E. P. Dutton.

Bloomfield, K. (1993). A comparison of alcohol consumption between lesbians and heterosexual women in an urban population, *Drug and Alcohol Dependency, 33,* 257-69.

Bonilla, L. and Porter, J. (1990). A comparison of Latino, black and non-Hispanic white attitudes toward homosexuality. *Hispanic Journal of Behavioral Sciences, 12* (4), 437-452.

Bradford, J. and Ryan, C. (1988) *The national lesbian health care survey: Final report.* Washington DC: National Lesbian/Gay Health Foundation.

Breeze. (1985). Social service needs and resources in rural communities. In H. Hidalgo, T. Peterson, and N. Woodman (Eds.), *Lesbian and gay issues: A resource manual for social workers* (pp. 43-48). Silver Spring, MD: National Association of Social Workers.

Cass, V. (1979). Homosexual identity formation: A theoretical model. *Journal of Homosexuality, 4*(3), 219-237.

Chan, C. (1989). Issues of identity development among Asian-American lesbians and gay men. *Journal of Counseling & Development, 68*(1), 16-20.

Chu, S., Bushler, J., Fleming, P., and Berkelman, R. (1990). Epidemiology of reported cases of AIDS in lesbians, United States 1980-89. *American Journal of Public Health, 80*(11), 1380-1381.

Clunis, D. M. and Green, G. D. (1993) *Lesbian couples: Creating healthy relationships for the 90's.* Seattle: Seal Press.

Cochron, S. and Mays, V. (1988) The Black Woman's Relationship Project: A National Survey of Black Lesbians. In W. Scott and M. Shernoff (Eds.), *The Source Book on Lesbian and Gay Health Care* (pp. 55-56). Washington, DC: National Lesbian/Gay Health Foundation.

DeCrescenzo, T. (Ed.). (1994). Helping gay and lesbian youth: New policies, new programs, new practice. [Special Issues]. *Journal of Gay and Lesbian Social Services, 1*(3/4).

Deevy, S. (1990). Older women: An invisible minority. *Journal of Gerontological Nursing, 16*(5), 35-39.

Deniston, K. (1989). Alcohol awareness. *Our Voice, 4*(1), 1.

DeStefano, G. (1986, June 24). Gay drug abuse. *The Advocate,* (449), 42-47.

Division of HIV/AIDS Prevention. (1996). *Report on lesbian HIV issues meeting April, 1995.* 1-14.

Dorfman, R., Walters, K., Burke, P., Hardin, L., Karanik, T., Raphael, J., and Silverstein, E. (1995). Old, sad, and alone: The myth of the aging homosexual. *Journal of Gerontological Social Work, 24*(1/2), 29-44.

Dworkin, J. and Kaufer, D. (1995). Social services and bereavement in the gay and lesbian community. In G. Lloyd and M. A. Kuszelewicz (Eds.), *HIV Disease: Lesbians, gays, and the social service.* Binghamton, NY: Harrington Park Press.

Freud, S. (1987). Letter to an American mother. *Homosexuality and American Psychiatry.* In R. Bayer (Ed.), Princeton University Press (Letter originally written 1935), p. 27.

Garnets, L., Herek, G., and Levy, B. (1992). Violence and victimization of lesbians and gay men: Mental health consequences. In G. Herek and K. Berrill (Eds.), *Hate Crimes* (pp. 207-226). Newbury Park, CA: Sage.

Germain, C. B. (1981). The ecological approach to people-environment transactions. *Social Casework: The Journal of Contemporary Social Work, 62,* 323-333.

Germain, C.B. and Gitterman, A. (1996). *The life model of social work practice, second edition.* New York: Columbia University Press.

Green, R. (1978). Sexual identity of 37 children raised by homosexual or transexual parents. *American Journal of Psychiatry, 135*(6), 696

Grier, B. and Cassidy, C. (1995). *The first time ever.* Tallahassee, FL: The Naiad Press.

Gunter, P. (1988). Rural gay men and lesbians in need of services and understanding. In M. Shernoff and W. Scott (Eds.), *The sourcebook on lesbian/gay health care,* second edition (pp. 49-53). Washington, DC: National Lesbian/Gay Health Foundation.

Hall, M. (1978). Lesbian families: Cultural and clinical issues. *Social Work, 23*(5), 31-35.

Hammond, N. (1989). Lesbian victims of relationship violence. In E. Cole and E. Rothblum (Eds.), *Loving boldly: Issues facing lesbians* (pp. 89-105). Binghamton, NY: Harrington Park Press.

Hansen, E. (1995). *Report on lesbian HIV issues meeting April 1995.* Atlanta: Center for Disease Control and Prevention.

Hart, B. (1986). Lesbian battering: An examination. In K. Lobel (Ed.), *Naming the violence: Speaking out about lesbian battering* (pp. 231-260). Seattle: Seal Press.

Hidalgo, H. (Ed.). (1995). Lesbians of color: Social and human services. [Special Issue]. *Journal of Gay and Lesbian Social Services, 3*(2).

Johnson, S., Smith, E., and Guether, S. (1987). Comparison of gynecologic care problems between lesbians and bisexual women: A survey of 2,345 women. *Journal of Reproductive Medicine,*(32), p. 805.

Kehoe, M. (1989). *Lesbians over 60 speak for themselves.* Binghamton, NY: Harrington Park Press.

Kirkpatrick, M., Smith, C., and Roy, R. (1981). Lesbian mothers and their children: A comparative survey. *American Journal of Orthopsychiatry, 51*(3), 545-551.

Kurdek, L. A. (Ed.). (1994). Social services for gay and lesbian couples. [Special Issue]. *Journal of Gay and Lesbian Social Services, 1*(2).

Kus, R. J. (Ed.). (1995). Addiction and recovery in gay and lesbian persons. [Special Issue]. *Journal of Gay and Lesbian Social Services, 2*(1).

Lewis, S. (1979). *Sunday's women.* Boston: Beacon Press.

Lloyd, G. A. and Kuszelewicz, M. A. (Eds.). (1995). HIV disease: Lesbians, gays and the social services. [Special Issue]. *Journal of Gay and Lesbian Social Services, 2*(3/4).

Lobel, S. (1986). *Naming the violence: Speaking out about lesbian battering.* Seattle: Seal Press.

Lovinger, R. (1994). Religious issues. In J. Rouch, W. Van Orum, and N. Stilwell (Eds.), *The counseling source book: A practical reference on contemporary issues* (pp. 202-222). New York: Crossroad.

Martin, A. (1991). Power of empathic relationships: Bereavement therapy with a lesbian widow. In C. Silverstein (Ed.), *Gays, lesbians, and their therapists* (pp.172-186). New York: W.W. Norton and Co.

McDonald, H. and Steinhorn, A. (1993). *Understanding homosexuality: A guide for those who know, love or counsel gay and lesbian individuals,* New York: Crossroad.

McKirnan, D. and Peterson, P. (1989). Alcohol and drug use among homosexual men and women: Epidemiology and population characteristics. *Addictive Behavior,* (14), 545-553.

Nelson, J. B. (1985). Religious and moral issues in working with homosexual clients. In J. Gonsiorek (Ed.), *A guide to psychotherapy with gay and lesbian clients* (pp. 163-175). Binghamton, NY: Harrington Park Press.

NiCarthy, G. (1982). *Getting free: You can end abuse and take back your life.* Seattle: Seal Press.

NiCarthy, G. (1987). *The ones who got away: Women who left abusive partners.* Seattle: Seal Press.

O'Hanlon, K. A. (1995). Lesbian health and homophobia: Perspectives for the treating obstetrician gynecologist. *Current Problems in Obstetrics, Gynecology and Fertility, 4*(18), 93-136.

Peterson, K. J. (Ed.) (1996). Health care for lesbians and gay men: Confronting homophobia and heterosexism. [Special Issue]. *Journal of Gay and Lesbian Social Services, 5*(1).

Pies, C. (1985). *Considering parenthood: A workbook for lesbians.* San Francisco: Spinsters Ink.

Quam, J. K. (Ed.) (1997). *Social services for older gay men and lesbians.* Binghamton, NY: The Haworth Press.

Rafkin, L. (1990). *Different mothers.* San Francisco: Cleis Press Inc.

Renzetti, C. M. and Miley, C. H. (Eds.). (1996). Violence in gay and lesbian domestic partnerships. [Special Issue]. *Journal of Gay and Lesbian Social Services, 4*(1).

Rubin, N. (1981). Clinical issues with disabled lesbians. *Catalyst,* (12), 37-45.

Schneider, M. (1989). Sappho was a right-on adolescent. In G. Herdt (Ed.), *Gay and lesbian youth* (pp. 111-130). Binghamton, NY: The Haworth Press.

Schulenberg, J. (1985). *Gay parenting: A complete guide for gay men and lesbians with children.* New York: Anchor Press.

Simon, B. (1987). *Never married women.* Philadelphia: Temple University Press.

Spong, J. S. (1992). *Living in sin? A bishop rethinks human sexuality.* San Francisco: Harper.

Spong, J. S. (1994) *Rescuing the bible from fundamentalism: A bishop rethinks the meaning of scripture.* San Francisco: Harper.

Steinhorn, A. (1982). Lesbian mothers—The invisible minority: Role of the mental health worker. *Women and Therapy, 1*(4), 35-48.

Tafoya, T. and Rowell, R. (1988). Counseling gay and lesbian native Americans. In M. Shernoff and W. Scott (Eds.), *The sourcebook on lesbian/gay health care,* second edition (pp. 63-67). Washington, DC: National Lesbian/Gay Health Foundation.

Wyers, N., (1987). Homosexuality in the family: Lesbian and gay spouses. *Social Work, 32*(2), 144-145.

Chapter 6

Group Work Practice with Gay Men and Lesbians

George S. Getzel

The subject of group work with gay men and lesbians represents a new and much needed area for conceptualization and innovation in the provision of social work services. This chapter will examine the nature of group work and its relevance to issues facing gay men, lesbians, and others struggling with sexual orientation and human sexuality.

The literature on the use of groups will be examined for its general emphases. A practice framework that encompasses social work with groups and services to gays and lesbians will be presented. Emerging practice principles for engagement and problem solving through groups will be detailed through case illustrations.

SOCIETAL CONTEXT

Group work practice is always a reflection of the historical and social context in which we live; this realization stands out boldly as the subject of services to the gay and lesbian communities is approached. This also makes the topic of this chapter both daunting and exciting.

In the last twenty-five years, unquestioned truths and received beliefs about homosexuality and those persons who have identified

---

In honor of Michael Shernoff and in loving memory of Diego Lopez and Kevin Mahony.

themselves as gay men and lesbians have undergone epic transformations that have profoundly touched the consciousness of
peoples throughout the world (Bell and Weinberg, 1978; Martin and
Dean, 1990; Nardi, Sanders, and Marmor, 1994). Beginning in
1969 with New York City's Stonewall Rebellion, a massive human
rights movement has commenced with rapidly growing effects on
human consciousness about sexuality, culture, politics, social relationships, and economics. In short, it is not only persons in the
struggle for self-identification as gay men and lesbians who have
been affected by social and historical changes, but millions of other
people throughout the world.

It would not be hyperbole to say that in many parts of the globe
the definition of what is "human" is being seriously challenged by
the quest for rights by gay men and lesbians. Any serious examination of the variety and the plasticity of human sexuality draws
deeply felt reactions from large numbers of people, particularly in
the case of homosexuality long stigmatized by the force of custom,
religious belief, and legal penalty (Foucault, 1978).

Fair employment, same-gender marriages, "gay bashing," the
plight of gay youth in high schools, and the right to custody and to
adopt children are among the growing number of subjects that
captured the attention of mass media and political candidates. Jux-
tapose this array of issues with the experiences of someone growing
up in the 1950s, when an average high school student could not
imagine that he or she could possibly be a friend of someone engaged in homosexual behaviors or be identified as a homosexual;
where the "closet" was the only conceivable place a person had to
maintain security in domestic and work life, in a world bereft of any
positive gay or lesbian role models to point out a direction and give
a vision of positive well-being (Nardi, Sanders, and Marmor, 1994).

In this societal context, group work finds numerous challenges in
the days ahead. Social workers with groups have an important
contribution to make by introducing groups that are gay and lesbian
affirmative, embodying humanistic values that place the human
being as the highest value and that affirm personal and cultural
diversity (Silo, 1994). Social workers, gay or straight, in their own
way must examine their own interior landscape—those experiences
early taught which may interfere with full and meaningful engage-

ment of gay men and lesbians in groups and the examination of human sexuality in groups of all kinds (Kooden, 1994; Morson and McInnis, 1983). Without a doubt, the vicissitudes of actual human sexual expression will grow larger as a subject of inquiry in groups of all kinds (Auerbach, 1985; Dunne, 1987; Weinberg, Williams, and Pryor, 1994).

MERITS OF GROUP WORK

The literature on group work directed toward gay men and lesbian women, detailed shortly, weighs heavily on services termed "group psychotherapy"—the earliest focusing on curing homosexuality (Conlin and Smith, 1982) rather than focusing on treating gays and lesbian clients for anxiety related to the coming-out process (Morrow, 1993; Morson and McInnis,1983), preexisting mental illness (Ball, 1994), alcoholism and substance abuse (Anderson and Henderson, 1985; Picucci, 1992; Ratner, 1993), domestic violence (Margolies and Leeder, 1995), and special circumstance of HIV/AIDS (Gambe and Getzel, 1989). Short of the fruitless and demeaning goal of curing homosexuality, more contemporary treatment emphases certainly have their value but do not adequately address the conceptual underpinnings of groups and their special merit for gay men and lesbians as fully realized human beings.

Treatment models, whether directed at gay men or lesbians, subsume an objectifying epistemology (Schwartz, 1976) of which oppressed people seeking help are justifiably wary. The shadow of the medical model in the guise of a new or an old white coat is and should be a source of concern for social workers in their interactions with gay men and lesbians. The special challenge to group work practice is to abet a group process that focuses on maximizing the potential for growth, belonging, and health as group members reach out to each other and to a world that extends beyond the boundaries of the group (Schwartz, 1961). An essential interactionist perspective (Schwartz, 1976) favors the strengths of group members and the interactions of people as they find common ground and overcome the obstacles that intrude from within and without.

At its best, a group work approach identifies the group as a need-meeting arrangement in which members together identify those activities that will maximize their functioning in the group and in the world that surrounds them. The worker seeks to maximize the power of the group as whole and members begin to identify concerns that affect their social relations and activities.

Mutual aid, the assistance members provide each other, is the special resource of groups (Gitterman and Shulman, 1994). Members learn about themselves and through the example of others; they discover the commonalities of their situations and feel the solidarity of peers and their expressions of altruism. The positive achievements of other group members provide guidance and instill hope about success in the future. The pains of human existence find a safe arena for exploration and acceptance (Yalom, 1975, 1993).

LITERATURE REVIEW

The literature on group work for gay men and lesbians is very limited, as is the case of the broader behavioral sciences literature. The bulk of the literature in recent years in social work and other disciplines has emphasized the importance of groups for the treatment of gay men with AIDS (Gambe and Getzel, 1989; Getzel and Mahony, 1990; Getzel, 1991a, b), and in one case lesbian women who are HIV positive (Foster, Stevens, and Hall, 1994). Educational groups for HIV preventions among gay men began to appear in the late 1980s (Palacios-Jímenez and Shernoff, 1986).

Significantly, there have been some important recent formulations by social worker on group services directed to gay men (Ball and Lipton, 1997) and on lesbians focusing on the coming-out process (Englehardt, 1997; Morrow, 1996). The use of groups with adolescents has also been noted (Morrow, 1993). A dearth of literature exists on gay and lesbian aging and group work intervention, although there are increasing larger cohorts of older gay men (Dawson, 1982; Getzel, in press) and lesbians (Adelman, 1991) who are sharing a unique socialization process that they bring to their later years. Life review groups for these cohorts are a promising area of intervention.

A GROUP WORK APPROACH

Group work services to gay men, lesbians, and others should have potential to deepen and to enrich the extant informal supports.

The natural informal supports of peers, friends, neighbors, and kin in the gay and lesbian community provide a vital source of positive pride (Adelman, 1991; Hart et al., 1990). Services to youth, the aging, as well as community centers offering an array of programs are growing significantly in urban geographic centers where there are large gay and lesbian populations. The presence of self-help groups such as Gay Alcoholic's Anonymous are also vital resources, which alongside of gay and lesbian parent support groups bear special recognition as evidence of extant groups in communities.

Groups with professional leadership also have an important role to play, as evidenced by the hundreds of support groups throughout this country and the world providing services to gay men with AIDS and their caregivers (Getzel, 1997). The model for this form of service delivery began when gay and bisexual men and lesbians created the first services to people with AIDS.

Central to the use of groups in the gay community is group work's efficacy in handling the individual's relationship with "the other" in the group and outside the boundaries of the group prompted by circumstances related to *identity issues, crisis situations,* and *existential conditions.* The calling forth of the group as a vehicle of support and problem solving becomes persuasive and powerful if one or more of these circumstances exist in the experience of people to be served.

The contemporary circumstances of many gay men and lesbians lend themselves to the use of groups to address the practical issues associated with the management of identity issues, crises related to conditions of bias and oppression, and existential conditions that press the individual to seek meaning in the face of oppression, loneliness, and prospect of death. For example, the problems of AIDS for gay men, of adolescent suicide for gay youth, and of negative anticipations in later life may present special challenges to gay men and lesbians at different points in the life cycle.

This approach of examining problems of living geared to gay men and lesbians can be generalized to all human beings. And well it should be, since the divisions that society makes between gay men and lesbians and the rest of the population are becoming more indecipherable, confused, and unclear (Barringer, 1993; Homosexual attraction, 1994). The problems of gay men and lesbians reflect the circumstances of *all* people trying to manage the vicissitudes of daily existence in society with all of the attendant obstacles of accident and human interference that create pain and suffering.

CASE ILLUSTRATIONS

The following are examples of social work practice with a humanistic perspective. Principles for group work practice with gay men, lesbians, and others are introduced through the illustrations. While in no way exhaustive of the array of *circumstances* that merit group work activity, they represent a beginning effort to look systematically at general group work principles for serving gay men and lesbians.

Identity Issues

Identity issues may occur in a group when members handle the arduous dual processes of coming to a personal recognition of sexual interests, self-identifications, and self-revealing a sexual identity to significant others. The following case illustration presents the dynamics of a support group of lesbians who seek mutual support in managing the day-to-day issues of being "out" as lesbians in the community. The group takes place in a women's center in an urban neighborhood with a large concentration of lesbians.

A social worker, a self-identified lesbian, is leading a support group of professional women twenty-eight through forty-seven years old, a few of whom have been married to men and are now in lesbian relationships. Others are at different stages of coming out to family and peers. This excerpt of group process begins with the expression of happiness by one group member in cementing her relationship with a partner, prompting a younger group member to speak about her loneliness and fear of coming out. The worker makes rich use of group feedback to maximize the sharing of different experiences about the uncertainties about committed relationships. Group members benefit from hearing each other's efforts to reconcile themselves to their emerging sexual orientation. The mutual aid of group members in addressing particular concerns of individuals builds a group culture of honesty and trust.

Alice excitedly tells the group that she and her partner just closed on their contract to buy a cooperative apartment. She sees this as an important point in their relationship—"almost like getting married." Jean, her partner, had been hesitant "to put all her money" into such a big investment. Over recent group sessions, Alice fretted about Jean's indecision as, perhaps, indicating Jean's lack of real love for her. Jean has been divorced from her husband for three years; Alice and she have been together for four years. While very devoted companions, Alice confided to group members her fear that Jean might abandon her for another person, "even her ex." While not shying away from Alice's concern, the group worker asks the group if they ever shared Alice's apprehensions about the solidity of their relationships with their partners. Some group members exchange stories of their recurrent fears, while searching out if there is any basis for Alice's worries.

Over the last few weeks, group members spoke about how hard the decision to come out was for them and the anxiety they have of losing their lover through abandonment, including death from breast cancer. Exploration into the details of her relationship give increasing reassurance to Alice that there is a solid base in her relationship with Jean. The group positively rejoices in the news about the co-op. The worker underlines the importance of the mutual aid that the group is able to offer Alice.

Amid the jubilance of the group, Denise, a younger member of the group, is seen as trying to smile but hiding her tears. Another group member asks her what is happening. Denise says that she does not want to ruin it for the Alice and the group. When pressed, Denise speaks about how upset she is for not coming out to her father after the Jewish holidays as she last discussed doing . . .

Crisis Situations

Group work has special benefits in helping persons handle both the emotional and instrumental issues that arise from crisis situations. Golan (1978) affirms that during a crisis, the individual faces a significant obstacle to achieving a specific life goal that is perceived to be insurmountable by otherwise satisfactory extant problem-solving ability.

The group becomes a context and means to assist group members mobilize available knowledge and mutual aid activity on behalf of overcoming serious obstacles interfering with life goals. In the following illustration, a group of gay and lesbian teenagers meet in a drop-in group. The group takes place in a multiservice agency which serves adolescents and which offers free health, mental health, and recreational services on a walk-in basis.

While the group has a core membership, it is open ended by design for gay, lesbian, bisexual, and transgender youth of different racial and ethnic backgrounds. The group has a social worker convening the group, and some of the older members of the group take on mentoring and "buddy" roles to other members in crisis.

In the group process excerpt, members assist one of their peers who has been subjected to bias and the threat of physical violence in a so-called "normal" high school:

> Julian comes to the group looking very depressed and unkempt, a significant change from his usual appearance. The group members seem to disregard him for the first fifteen minutes of the session, but become very somber when the group worker notes that Julian is uncharacteristically quiet. In defense of him, Mara angrily tells the worker that he will talk when and if wants to (as if the worker should mind his business). Mara seems to know what is up, as do other members of the group.
>
> Joseph breaks through the group's silence by attacking Mara for protecting Julian. Joseph says that, "Other guys will continue to attack Julian if he does not stand up for himself and quit acting like a fag. You look for trouble wearing eye makeup."
>
> Julian says that he regrets bothering the group, but cryptically indicates that no one should worry, because he intends to quit high school or "do something else." Several members become quite concerned and ask him what he means. The worker intervenes that he too is concerned not only with what Julian is saying, but how he is saying it.

Mara interjects he does not have to quit high school, but can make a transfer to the Harvey Milk High School for gay and lesbian youth. Julian breaks down in tears; he does not want to leave his current school, but cannot sleep at night and sometimes wishes he was born a girl. This initiates a long discussion in the group with some members also expressing similar feelings about dealing with the stress of being a gay or lesbian teen.

Existential Conditions

There is no greater imperative that is as persistently avoided by people in the course of their daily lives than bringing meaning to living. The routines and the compensations of momentary pleasure and diversions usually are varied and sufficient to prevent us from asking questions about the meaning and direction of our lives. The existential question at its core is, Why should I live? It is a question positively responded to by actions in the world that create meaning. Nothing is given a priori, but meaning is found by each human exercising his or her freedom or intentionality within the parameters of his or her existence. Pain and suffering in the world are the obstacles that each human being encounters, and it is the overcoming of such obstacles that renders meaning (Silo, 1994).

Gay men and lesbians face serious existential concerns. For example, the last decade-and-a-half of the AIDS pandemic has made us aware of the pain endured by the gay and lesbian communities caused by horrific illness and cumulative deaths of loved ones. A related existential condition is the suffering of gay men and lesbians rejected by families of origin because of their homosexuality. For gays and lesbians, homosexuality represents an intrinsic and ultimately positive expression of intimacy. The burden of rejection may be isolation and the incorporation of negative images of the self. Groups provide the sanctuary for discussing these pressing existential questions.

The following process excerpt of a support group of gay men diagnosed with AIDS illustrates the collision between the theme of dying, in this case prompted by the death of a group member, and the quest of surviving members to find meaning in living. The death of members, the development of disfiguring and disorienting symptoms, and shifts in their interpersonal relations create a life review process within the group. The group worker supports members' honest exchanges of painful material and encourages mutual aid and practical problem solving as members experience declines in functional capacity.

This is the first meeting since Joe's death and funeral. Joe had been a member of the group for nearly three years. His forbearance in the face of the spread of Kaposi's sarcoma lesions over his entire face and apparent HIV-related dementia have been subjects of recent discussion in the group. Group members were able to tell Joe of their deep admiration of him in overcoming successive health challenges, and his devotion to them was evidenced in his frequent phone calls to check in to see how other group members were doing after he was too ill to attend the group.

Doug says that while he admires Joe, he does not intend to draw out his dying, if he becomes severely sick. He refuses to humiliate himself and look foolish to others, especially if he becomes demented. Allan, with a slight smile on his face says, "Easier said than done."

Waiting out the group's silence, the group worker asks members what seems to be happening. Steven tells the worker it is nothing new between Doug and Allan, "They both 'turned on' each other by fighting."

Group members break out in uncontrollable laughter and engage in making sexualizing remarks. Doug says it is good to laugh about dying, and that he has even talked to his friends about his funeral. He wants to have a change of clothing twice during the viewing of his body. Doug explains, "In life, he always tries to be the life of the party, and in death he certainly does not intend to bore anyone to death."

Peter asks if one of his intended changes of outfit would be a fashionable dress, hat, and long gloves. The group again capitulates into laughter and many humorous asides. The worker acknowledges that it is important to have some relief after this difficult week.

Allan begins to speak about the beautiful eulogy Joseph's lover gave at the funeral. The group members exchange warm memories of Joe. Later in the session group members speak about updating "advanced directives"—granting medical decision making to a relative or a friend in the event they are unable to make medical decisions for themselves. This discussion is especially difficult for members whose closest family members and friends have withdrawn from them over the last few years.

DISCUSSION

Groups that deal with identity issues, crisis situations, and existential conditions are part of an array of much needed social work services that aim at fuller integration of gay men and lesbians into society. Groups that are gay and lesbian oriented are testing grounds and laboratories for its members to make decisions that enhance their quality of living and societal participation.

Of equal importance is the integration of gay men and lesbians into groups of so-called "straight" group members. All social workers must examine their internal landscape for ideas and attitudes that inhibit or enhance the discussion of human sexuality represented by each member of a group. In short, no assumptions can be made of a group member's sexual orientation, attitudes, and behaviors. This vital discussion of sexuality cannot occur until a feeling of trust is experienced about the group worker and a group culture is created that is open and relatively nonjudgmental.

The paucity of literature on human sexuality in social work and the effective indifference of social work education to the subject must be overcome in the years ahead. Practitioners in and outside the gay and lesbian communities must communicate areas of need and contribute their practice know-how to the literature and the extension of services to the gay and lesbian communities in different regions of the country and in urban, rural, and suburban settings.

Emerging practice with gay men and lesbians offers vital insights to social work with groups with all vulnerable populations. Members of a group fully benefit from the experience when universal questions of meaning about being a human being are explored: Who am *I* in terms of the *other?* How do I move in the direction of greater coherence between my thoughts, beliefs, and actions? How do I overcome the crises associated with living in the world that challenge personal coherence? What must I do to express my own personal diversity and accept personal and social diversity in others? And ultimately, do I want to live and if so how?

REFERENCES

Adelman, M. (1991). Stigma, gay lifestyles and adjustment to aging: A study of late-life gay men and lesbians. *Journal of Homosexuality, 20*(3/4), 7-32.

Anderson, S. C. and Henderson, D. C. (1985). Working with lesbian alcoholics. *Social Work, 30*(6), 518-525.

Auerbach, S. (1985). Groups for wives of gay and bisexual men. *Social Work, 3*(4), 321-325.

Ball, S. (1994). A group model for gay and lesbian clients with chronic mental illness. *Social Work, 39*(1), 109-115.

Ball S. and Lipton, B. (1997). Group work with gay men. In P. Ephross and G. Grief (Eds.), *Group work with populations at risk* (pp. 259-277). Oxford: Oxford University Press.

Barringer, F. (1993 April 15). Sex survey of American men find 1% are gay. *The New York Times,* pp. 1, 18.

Bell, A. P. and Weinberg, M. S. (1978), *Homosexualities: A study of diversity among men and women.* New York: Simon and Schuster.

Conlin, D. and Smith, J. (1982). Group psychotherapy for gay men. *Journal of Homosexuality, 7*(2/3), 105-112.

Dawson, K. (1982 November). Serving the older gay community. *Siecus Report,* 5-6.

Dunne, E. J. (1987). Helping gay fathers come out to their children. *Journal of Homosexuality, 14*(3/4), 213-222.

Englehardt, B. J. (1997). Group work with lesbians. In P. Ephross and G. Grief (Eds.), *Group work with populations at risk* (pp. 278-291). Oxford: Oxford University Press.

Foster, S. B., Stevens, E. P., and Hall, J. M. (1994). Offering support group services for lesbians living with HIV. *Women in Therapy, 15*(2), 69-83.

Foucault, M. (1978). *The history of sexuality: An introduction, Vol. I,* New York: Vintage Books.

Gambe, R. and Getzel, G. S. (1989). Group work with gay men with AIDS. *Social Casework, 70*(3), 172-179.

Getzel, G. S. (1991a). AIDS. In A. Gitterman (Ed.), *Handbook of social work with vulnerable populations* (pp. 35-64). New York: Columbia University Press.

Getzel, G. S. (1991b). Survival modes of people with AIDS in groups. *Social Work, 36*(1), 7-11.

Getzel, G. S. (1997). Group work practice with people with AIDS. In P. Ephross and G. Grief (Eds.), *Group work with populations at risk* (pp. 42-55). Oxford: Oxford University Press.

Getzel, G. S. (in press). Gay men in later life. In L. Kaye and J. Kosberg (Eds.), *Elderly men: Special problems and challenges.* New York: Springer.

Getzel, G. S. and Mahony, K. (1990). Confronting human finitude: Group work with people with AIDS. *Journal of Gay and Lesbian Psychotherapy, 1*(3), 105-120.

Gitterman, A. and Shulman, L. (1994). The life model, mutual aid, oppression, and the mediating function. In A. Gitterman and L. Shulman (Eds.), *Mutual aid groups, vulnerable populations and the life cycle* (pp. 3-28). New York: Columbia University Press.

Golan, N. (1978). *Treatment in crisis situations.* New York: Free Press.

Hart, G., Fitzpatrick, R., McLean, J., Dawson, J., and Boulton, M. (1990). Gay men, social support, HIV disease: A study of social integration of the gay community. *AIDS Care, 2,* 163-170.

Homosexual attraction is found in 1 of 5. (1994 September 6). *The New York Times,* p. 14.

Kooden, H. (1994). The gay male therapist as an agent of socialization. *Journal of Gay and Lesbian Psychotherapy, 2*(2), 39-65.

Margolies, L. and Leeder, E. (1995). Violence at the door: Treatment of lesbian batterers. *Violence Against Women, 1*(2), 139-157.

Martin, J. L. and Dean, L. (1990). Developing a community sample of gay men for an epidemiologic study of AIDS. *American Behavioral Scientist, 33,* 546-561.

Morrow, D. F. (1993). Social work with gay and lesbian adolescents. *Social Work, 38*(6), 655-660.

Morrow, D. F. (1996). Coming-out issues for adult lesbians: A group intervention. *Social Work, 40*(6), 647-656.

Morson, T. and McInnis, R. (1983). Sexual identity issues in group work: Gender, social sex role, and sexual orientation considerations. *Social Work with Groups, 6*(3/4), 67-77.

Nardi, P. M., Sanders, D., and Marmor, J. (1994). *Growing up before Stonewall: Life histories of some gay men.* London: Routledge.

Palacios-Jimenez, L. and Shernoff, M. (1986). *Erotizing safer sex.* New York: Gay Men's Health Crisis.

Picucci, M. (1992). Planning an experiential weekend workshop for lesbians and gay males in recovery. *Journal of Chemical Dependency Treatment, 5*(1), 119-139.

Ratner, E. F. (1993). Treatment issues for chemically dependent lesbians and gay men. In L. D. Garnets and D. C. Kimmel (Eds.), *Psychological perspectives on lesbian and gay male experiences* (pp. 567-558), New York: Columbia University.

Schwartz, W. (1961). The social worker in the group. In W. Schwartz (Ed.), *New perspectives on services to groups: Theory, organization and practice* (pp. 7-34). New York: National Association of Social Workers.

Schwartz, W. (1976). Between client and system: Mediating function. In R. Roberts and H. Northen (Eds.), *Theories of social work with groups* (pp. 171-197). New York: Columbia University Press.

Silo. (1994). *Letters to my friends: On the social and personal crisis in today's world.* San Diego: Latitude Press.

Weinberg, M. S., Williams, C. J., and Pryor, D. W. (1994). *Dual attraction: Understanding bisexuality.* New York: Oxford University Press.

Yalom, I. (1975). *The theory and practice of group psychotherapy,* second edition. New York: Basic Books.

Yalom, I. (1993). *The theory and practice of group psychotherapy,* fourth edition. New York: Basic Books.

Chapter 7

Social Work Practice with Gay Men and Lesbians Within Families

Gerald P. Mallon

The emergence of gay men and lesbians as a community that has begun to name and claim its right to be viewed within the context of family systems is a relatively recent phenomenon. Although gay and lesbian persons are frequently and fallaciously portrayed by some in the media and by many politicians from the radical right as vehemently antifamily, nothing could be further from the truth. In fact, the truth is that families are important for gay and lesbian persons. Like all people, gay men and lesbians don't appear magically in the world but have parents, siblings, and other extended family members. Families supply physical and emotional sustenance, connect individuals with their pasts, and provide a context within which people learn about the world, including attitudes and mores of society (Berzon, 1992). Gay and lesbian persons need to be part of their families as much as any other people. Given the stigmatizing status that homosexuality still holds for many in society, the family is one place where a gay or lesbian person most needs to feel accepted. Oftentimes, however, this is not the case as it is not the gay or lesbian individual who rejects his or her family, but family members who reject and disown him or her simply because of his or her gay or lesbian sexual orientation.

All gay and lesbian persons grow up within a family context, which in most cases is usually heterosexual and heterocentric. Viewed within an ecological framework, being a gay or lesbian person within a heterosexual family is by its very nature a transactional process that is generally not a "good-fit"—unless the family is not antigay and antilesbian. Having to keep secret one's sexual identity and affectional preferences creates stresses that are the result not of the individual's gay or lesbian identity but of Western society's antigay/lesbian attitudes. Living within or being a member of a family system where one cannot be or articulate who they truly are places gay and lesbian persons in a constant state of having to negotiate life within environments that are oftentimes hostile to their existence. Slater's (1995) recent work concurs, noting that much of what is known about family life cycles is largely irrelevant to the experiences of gay men and lesbians since it is predicated on the idea of a heterosexual couple at the center and a family bonded by blood or marriage. Since none of these conditions exist in the lives of gay men and lesbians, social workers who work with clients who are other than heterosexually oriented must be conscious of this distinction.

Social workers preparing to practice with gay men and lesbians within the context of their family systems need to acknowledge that these clients will present at any social service or health care agency, in private practice seeking direct or clinical social work services, and in any of the field of practice areas. These men and women may be at any stage of the life cycle, and it is important that social workers do not make any assumptions about the nature of these clients and their families or their presenting problems prior to doing a complete psychosocial assessment with a detailed family history.

Competent social work practice with gay and lesbian persons within the family context draws on an exceptionally broad and diverse body of knowledge. Family-based practice with gay and lesbian persons and their family is complex. Thus, in order to successfully intervene with this population, social workers must, as Laird (1996, p. 117) points out, "be able to bracket and move beyond [their] own prior understandings and assumptions that probably have been shaped in a heterosexist and homophobic context." Social workers should also become familiar with the available literature, which broadly addresses the common clinical issues that pertain to lesbians, gay men, and their families (Allen and Demo, 1995; Brown, 1988; Laird, 1983, 1996; Lui and Chan, 1996; Preston, 1992).

Drawing on the literature, theories, concepts, and models that are most commonly used to inform and guide social work practice with families, this chapter is limited to an analysis of the gay and lesbian person within the context of their family system and examines the primary reciprocal exchanges and transactions that lesbian and gay persons and their families face as they confront the unique person:environment tasks involved in a society that assumes all of its members are heterosexual. Consequently, this chapter explores the following three areas: (1) the experiences of gay men and lesbians within the context of their families of origin; (2) the experiences of gay men and lesbians who elect to become parents and thus create their own families; and (3) the prominence of families of creation (where lesbians and gay men share their lives with other gay men, lesbian, or heterosexually-oriented nonrelatives to develop a support network of nonrelated persons that acts as a family) within the lives of gay men and lesbians.

DEFINITION OF FAMILY

Despite the increasing emphasis on family-centered social work practice (Hartman and Laird, 1983) there is a tendency for practitioners to view gay and lesbian persons primarily, if not solely, as individuals rather than as members of a family of origin and as possible creators of their own family systems (either families of choice or biological families) at a later point in their lives. By not acknowledging that "human beings can be understood and helped only in the context of the intimate and powerful human systems of which they are a part," of which the family is one of the most important (Hartman and Laird, 1983, p. 4), practitioners may miss out on many important opportunities for fostering more positive relationships between gay and lesbian persons and their families.

One definition of family emphasizes the coming together to meet needs as one criterion: "A family becomes a family when two or more individuals have decided they are a family that in the intimate here-and-now environment in which they gather, there is a sharing of the emotional needs for closeness, of living space which is deemed 'home,' and of those roles and tasks necessary for meeting the biological, social, and psychological requirements of the individuals involved" (Hartman and Laird, 1983, p. 30). Rothberg and Weinstein (1996, p. 57) suggest that we consider the following examples: two adults of the same gender living together within the same habitat or in separate habitats who identify as partners; gay, lesbian, bisexual individuals and their heterosexual parents, siblings, grandparents, aunts, uncles, cousins, and other relatives; same-gendered couples or gay, lesbian, or bisexual individuals who are rearing children; same gendered couples and a former spouse (either heterosexual or gay or lesbian) and their children; heterosexually married couples in marriages where one or both spouses have same-gendered relationships apart from their marriages; a group of nonrelated gay, lesbian, or bisexual persons living together as a family of creation; and many other combinations of families limited only by the limits of the participant's inventiveness.

Even though society often stereotypes homosexually oriented individuals as Caucasian, effeminate men; the family configurations of lesbian, gay, and bisexual persons include people from every ethnic, social, economic, racial, cultural, and religious background. The issues for gay, lesbian, and bisexual people of color communities are both diverse and complex, as cultural, racial, religious, power, and privilege issues and social and psychological themes intersect. Although these issues were fully explored by Walters in the third chapter of this text, these concerns have special significance with respect to family dynamics (Carter and McGoldrick, 1989). Consider the following case example:

> Mary is a nineteen-year-old college student who lives at home with her mother, father, and two younger male siblings. Mary's mother, who lives with a chronic disease, multiple sclerosis, works full-time and is the primary nurturer in the family system. Mary's father is an accountant in a large firm in an urban area and works long hours; he is largely unavailable to his family, investing his energy in his job. The family identifies culturally and racially as African American, is socioeconomically middle class, and is staunchly Baptist. Mary has just completed her second year at a local community college and has been on the Dean's List for all four semesters. She has always been the family's most distinguished student and has always been viewed as helpful and caring by both her parents

and her brothers. Recently, however, she met a woman at her school, and after several dates, they entered into an intimate relationship. This is the first serious relationship for Mary, who has also in the past dated young men, and the second for her partner, who is two years older. Mary's mother is very concerned that she and her new "friend" are spending so much time together. Mary has always had a positive relationship with her mother, but she is afraid that coming out to her will change their relationship, particularly because her mother is devoted to the Baptist Church and because she has always frowned upon "those people." Not being able to be honest about her life is stressful and difficult for Mary, but she is unwilling to take a chance that her family will reject her if she comes out. As an adaptive measure, Mary has become increasingly distant from her family and secretive about her life and her relationship. This is a significant change for this family system which previously had perceived itself as a close-knit unit. Everyone in the family realizes that there have been serious changes within the family system, but no one talks about it.

From this brief sketch, one can begin to see how and why this is a family systems imbroglio. There are numerous stresses in this environment. The economy requires that the mother works to support her family despite her chronic illness; the young woman has been overcompensating for her hidden identity by excelling in academics and by trying to be the perfect child, while at the same time struggling in silence with her own emerging lesbian identity. Add to this case the racial, cultural, and religious factors in that the African-American culture and the Baptist church have irrefutable negative views of individuals (even family members) who are homosexually oriented and the fact that the young woman was fearful of disclosure. With these factors in mind it is not difficult to see why this family is a system that is at an impasse. As this case example suggests, many personal, family, and environmental factors converge and interact with each other to influence the family. In other words, human behavior is not solely a function of the person or the environment, but of the complex interaction between them.

AN ECOLOGICAL PERSPECTIVE

Ecology is the science that examines the relationship between living systems and their environments and has furnished a fitting metaphor for the ecological perspective of social work practice (Germain, 1979, 1991; Germain and Gitterman, 1980, 1996; Hartman and Laird, 1983; Meyer, 1983, 1988, 1993). Since all families live within the context of and are continually interacting with physical, social, and cultural environments, utilizing an ecological perspective of social work practice to work with gay and lesbian persons and families offers a broad conceptual lens for viewing family functioning and needs. Such a perspective requires frequent, ongoing transactions with multiple, complex systems, transactions through which both the family and the other systems are changed with consequences for both. Hess and Jackson (1995, p. 132) spell it out precisely when they say,

> When the consequences for family functioning undermine family functioning or integrity, and increase stress for the family members, or deplete the family's resources, social work intervention may be focused on the family, on the environmental system or systems, or on the transactions between them.

It is the reciprocal nature of these interactions, indeed, the purposeful intervention which one calls upon to improve the reciprocity in the exchange between family and its environment and which is at the core of the ecological perspective of social work practice with families.

The work of Germain and Gitterman (1980, 1996), draws on several sets of ecological concepts, including (1) exchange or transaction; (2) person:environment fit, adaptedness, and adaptation; (3) life stressors, stress, and coping; (4) relatedness, competence, self-concept, self-esteem, and self-direction; (5) vulnerability, oppression, abuse or misuse of power, social or technological pollution; (6) habitat and niche; and (7) life course. All are concepts which form the current theoretical foundation of what Germain and Gitterman (1996, p. 5) term "the life-model of social work practice" and which serve as the theoretical framework for this paper.

As lesbian, gay, and bisexual persons strive for the best person:environment "fit," many find, as a consequence of their environment's intolerance, that the fit is not good. Utilizing an ecological perspective, this author proposes an approach that suggests that gay and lesbian persons have three strategies of adaptation from which they may choose. A gay or lesbian person may actively decide to adapt to his or her environment's intolerance by attempting to change him or herself. (The gay or lesbian person might try to date or marry opposite-gendered individuals in an effort to change.) Or, they may attempt to modify their environment (by looking for cues within the various environments that signal that it is safe to disclose or at least to explore these options). Finally, some gay or lesbian persons may migrate to a new environment that could provide safety and sustain them with the nutrients necessary for health. (Individuals might leave their families of origin to seek other habitats or look for opportunities outside of their geographic environments, usually in urban areas, to locate cultural niches with others who are like them.) Consequently, practitioners need to seek to influence the direction of change within both the individual and his or her environment. With respect to the gay or lesbian person within a heterosexual family context, practitioners will interface with clients who are at every stage of this process. Some will continue to attempt to change themselves; others will continue to work toward changing their environments by educating families and assisting them in dealing with antigay and lesbian attitudes; others will distance themselves, physically and/or psychologically from their families, migrating to habitats that are perceived to be more affirming of their sexual orientation; others will adapt by creating their own families.

GAYS AND LESBIANS IN THE CONTEXT OF THEIR FAMILIES OF ORIGIN

Although the family relationships of gay men and lesbians are much more complex than characterized by numerous dynamics and issues than just one's disclosure to family members, it is disclosure of one's gay or lesbian identity to family members that seems to be the most central theme in both the literature and in real-life clinical cases. Disclosure of one's gay or lesbian identity to one's family of origin can occur at any point during the life span development (Adair and Adair, 1978; Berger, 1982, 1984, Berzon, 1992; Dank, 1971; Hersch, 1991; Hetrick and Martin, 1987; Kehoe, 1988; Kimmel and Sang, 1995; Quam, 1997; Sullivan and Schneider, 1987). Disclosure of one's gay or lesbian sexual orientation can occur when a child discloses to a parent, to a sibling, to a grandparent, or to other relatives, or conversely, when a parent discloses his or her sexual orientation to a child or their spouse. In other cases, gay and lesbian persons choose not to disclose to their family throughout the entire course of their lifetime.

Although gay men and lesbians are commonly clustered sociologically as if they were one group, there are very distinct differences between gay men and lesbians. These differences are manifest from both a developmental perspective and from a personal identity perspective and may have more to do with gender role and gender-bound socialization norms than with sexual orientation (Gilligan, 1982). Based on her own observations about ongoing family of origin connections in the lives of lesbians, Laird (1996, pp. 117-118) suggests that the portrayal of gays and lesbians as separate and isolated from their families better reflects the experiences of gay men than of lesbians.

Brown (1988) raises a number of key clinical issues that she delineates as common patterns for gay men and lesbians who are addressing the issue of coming out to families of origin. These include (1) distancing, emotionally and/or geographically, from the family of origin (as evidenced in the case example illustrated above); (2) a tacit agreement between the individual and the family that no one will discuss the individual's personal life ("they know, but we don't talk about it"); and (3) disclosure to one parent or sibling who is supportive, with the understanding that the individual will not tell other family members. All of these adaptations make gay men and lesbians more vulnerable to stress and distress.

Laird (1996, p. 116) additionally suggests that coming out to one's family is much more than a simple verbal disclosure. Being lesbian or gay can be manifested in a number of ways behaviorally and verbally, in the family of origin and in other contexts. Ponse (1976, p. 331) observed, "The family's awareness of the gay self usually occurs through observation of cues rather than by direct disclosure. . . . " A family's response to its family members' gay or lesbian identity will mirror the way in which the family has addressed other family issues. Families who are inflexible concerning the rules and mores of behaviors will most likely have more trouble. Families who have a history of openly discussing sensitive or controversial topics will more likely have an easier time. Whichever the case, family members who openly disclose their sexual orientation add an important and distinctive element to the family system. Most gay men and lesbians have experienced pain, hurt, estrangement, and their families have experienced isolation, anger, confusion, and distress over their family member's gay or lesbian identity. But it is also possible for gay men and lesbians and their families to move beyond these difficulties and to forge a more or less satisfying ongoing relationship. Gay or lesbian individuals must deal with their family's heterocentrism and their own, and family members must decide how they will support one another against a backdrop of marginality that they might never have anticipated.

DISCLOSURE TO FAMILIES OF ORIGIN

Most gay and lesbian persons are reared by people who are heterosexual; consequently, most families have no prior preparation for dealing with their family member's gay or lesbian sexual orientation. Families primarily convey strong heterosexual messages; that is, that heterosexual relationships are the only valid and appropriate life goals. Consequently, most heterosexual persons grow up within a societal context that is understanding and supportive of their lives. As individuals become aware of their sexuality, most are supported by families who encourage and discuss dating and attraction to the opposite gender. In contrast, the individual who is gay or lesbian, by and large, does not have such environmental nourishment, as they lack familial and cultural role models. Additionally, since gay and lesbian persons are different from other members of their families, their socialization process—as contrasted with the socialization process that occurs within people-of-color communities where all of the members of the family unit are of color and have accordingly suffered the effects of marginalization and stigmatization—does not offer a nurturing environment for them to develop a pride in their culture and/or teach them adaptive behaviors for coping with oppression and discrimination. This socialization deficiency frequently leaves gay and lesbian individuals unprepared and ill-equipped to deal with a societally discredited status (Hetrick and Martin, 1987).

Although the bulk of the professional literature that addresses the issue of gay and lesbian persons and their families focuses on parental reaction to disclosure by a child, empirical evidence (D'Augelli and Hershberger, 1993, p. 433) suggests that most individuals do not first come out to their families. In fact, the majority of gay and lesbian people (73 percent), disclosed first to a friend. Mothers were first told only 7 percent of the time; fathers or both parents were told first 1 percent of the time.

DISCLOSURE TO PARENTS

Gay men and lesbians must manage disclosure issues on a daily basis as coming out is a process and not just a one-time event. Lesbian and gay individuals must decide when, how, and if they decide to disclose to a whole range of family members—parents, grandparents, brothers, sisters, aunts, uncles, cousins, nieces, and nephews. Nonetheless, it is parental reaction to the disclosure of homosexual orientation that can cause the most stress for gay and lesbian persons. Dealing with a family member's gay or lesbian identity can create stress, tension, and emotional problems, sometimes provoking a hostile reaction even in families that are generally supportive and open. While many families develop effective coping devices to adjust to their family member's disclosure, other families are completely unprepared and react in a very unpredictable and negative manner, which may lead to family system malfunctions.

Parental perceptions of their child's sense of differentness points to two common reactions, as identified by Strommen (1989). The first is that most parents, unfamiliar with homosexuality, apply their negative conceptions of gay and lesbian identity to their children. The second aspect of this parental perception is powerful feelings of guilt and failure. Rothberg and Weinstein (1996) add that they have found one of the biggest problems for families with a gay or a lesbian family member is embarrassment. Perhaps a more appropriate characterization of this process is that there is a range of responses to a family member's disclosure. This is best captured in this description by Rothberg and Weinstein:

> When a family member comes out there are a multitude of responses. At one end of the spectrum is acceptance, . . . but rarely, if ever, is this announcement celebrated. Take for example, the announcement a heterosexual person makes to his or her family of origin of an engagement to marry. This is usually met with a joyous response, a ritual part and many gifts. The lesbian and gay man does not receive this response. Instead, the coming out announcement is often met with negative responses which can range from mild disapproval to complete nonacceptance and disassociation. These responses, though usually accepted, cause considerable stress and pain for the lesbian and gay person seeking parental approval. (p. 81)

Some families, particularly families with strong religious convictions, may openly condemn homosexuality, unaware that their own child is lesbian or gay. Blumenfeld and Raymond (1988) note that families with strong religious convictions often support their views of their religion even against a family member. Personal biases, particularly cultural or religious biases that view homosexuality negatively, can make coming out to parents a painful experience for many people, as evidenced by this man's story:

> I'm thirty-five years old and I'm still afraid to come out to my parents. I grew up in a small town in upstate New York. There were no people whom I could determine that were gay or lesbian. We were Catholic so there was always a lot of antigay rhetoric in our home. I couldn't wait to get out of there. I went away to college and after college, I moved away to live in a city where I could live among people who were like me. My family could never accept the fact that I am gay. They are too religious and too narrow-minded because of that.

Although some families might not openly denounce homosexuality, "the absence of discussion sends a negative message"

(Browning, 1987, p. 48), as illuminated by this quotation from a client:

> In my family, my parents know, but we don't talk about it. That's our unspoken agreement. I can bring my dates to their home and all, but we just never talk about the fact that they are my dates and that I'm gay. Every once in a while, my father, even though he knows that I am gay will say—"Hey, when are you gonna give all this up and get married?" I guess he just doesn't get it.

Families provide many opportunities for their members to receive positive reinforcement, approval, and validation for their heterosexual orientation. Heterosexual individuals rarely have their identity itself challenged as unacceptable. What a lesbian or gay person fears most is that their families will reject their personhood and that it will result in the destruction of their relationship with them, as this thirty-two-year-old woman's story illustrates:

> After years of saying nothing, I went home to visit my mother and I decided to have the talk with her. I said, Mom, I guess you know, but I am a lesbian. She got very quiet and said she'd really rather not talk about it. The rest of my time at home was uncomfortably quiet. I tried to bring up the subject again before I left and she stopped me. She said, "I don't understand this, and I just don't want to talk about it." I left wondering if I had made a big mistake, maybe I should have just stayed quiet about it.

In some cases, it is not the child who comes out to the parent, but the parent who comes out to the child, as in this case example of a fifty-four-year-old lesbian:

> I had been divorced from my children's father for more than ten years, I dated men, some even seriously, but one day I just met this woman and I fell in love with her. I realized at that point that I was a lesbian and since I was sharing my life with this woman, I had to talk to my kids and let them know. I have three adult children, two girls and a boy. I sat with each of

them privately and I just told them that I had realized after many years that I was a lesbian. They all dealt with it very well. But they are adults, living their own lives, so . . . I expected that they would be all right with it. I often wonder how it would have been though if they were younger.

Although it is not often the norm, parental reaction to a family member's disclosure can also be a positive experience increasing the level of intimacy and honesty with parents, as confirmed by this young man's story:

My mom always knew. When we finally sat down and "had the talk" and I said, "Mom I have to talk to you," she said, "I know; you're gay, right?" I was so relieved. I asked her, "How did you know?" And my Mom said, "Honey, I always knew that you were different." I had heard from so many of my friends how terrible their experiences were and even though my mother and I have always had a positive relationship, I was scared that she would not be able to deal with me being gay and it would ruin everything.

Unfortunately, for most people, parental disclosure is not the positive experience that this individual had. For many, it is a negative experience that can include anger, denial, guilt, or insistence on therapy to "change" the person's orientation. Griffin, Wirth, and Wirth (1986) confirm that initial parental reactions to disclosure can include breaking contact with their child, trying to change their family member, ignoring the issue, or accepting reality.

In some cases, adolescents, in particular, may not have the opportunity to voluntarily disclose their sexual orientation as they are "found out" by family members who "discover" their "secret" (Mallon, in press b). In these cases, verbal harassment or physical abuse by family members, as represented by this person's story, are commonplace.

My mother found out that I was gay when she found gay magazines that I had hidden in my room. She went crazy, she started beating me, cursing at me, and kept asking me, "Why do you want to be gay? Why do you want to be a homo? Why do you want to be a faggot? Don't you want a family and don't you want to make me a proud mother?" I said I didn't want a family and I didn't want a wife and she slapped me across the face. Then she gave an extension cord to my stepfather and he took over and started beating me.

Young people who have experienced this level of violence from their families in relation to their coming out may not only require social work intervention, but out-of-home placement (Mallon, 1992, in press a) to separate them from their families until and only if a reconciliation can be arranged.

Although gay men and lesbians are increasingly open to disclosing their sexual orientation to their families, some individuals continue to hide their gay or lesbian identity from their families. Some gay people go to elaborate extremes to hide their identity, for example, having separate telephone lines installed with the agreement that one partner is never to answer the phone of the other person. Others, even those who have cohabitated for years, make certain that they have two separate bedrooms even though they sleep together in one. In some cases, gay and lesbian couples even hide things that they feel might "give away" their identity from family members who visit their home. Such adaptations have a negative impact on their self-esteem and on their relationship. Even though there may be many signs for families that point to their child's gay or lesbian identity, many families act as though they prefer to believe that their child is heterosexual.

Some parents may erroneously believe that it was their role modeling that determined their child's sexual orientation. "What did I do wrong?" is a common self-blaming refrain. Parents may also worry about being blamed by people in the community, others may worry that their dream of having grandchildren might never materialize. The latter of these concerns are increasingly irrelevant as many gay and lesbian persons have or will decide that their orientation has nothing to do with their desire to create a family and to rear children. The reality is, however, that when a member of the family system comes out, the entire system faces the challenge of coming out. In fact, DeVine (1984) suggested that when one member of the family comes out, the entire family is also forced to come out as well.

Most of the family of origin issues that bring gay men and lesbians into contact with social work practitioners are the same problems that anyone would bring—how to deal with an overbearing parent, how to deal with the aftermath of a childhood filled with physical or sexual abuse, how to deal with an aging parent, how to reconcile cultural differences between the families of two spouses, and level of spouse acceptance. There are distinctions, as well, that are unique to the gay and lesbian experience: a sibling who does not accept his or her brother or sister's gay or lesbian life; a parent who has heretofore had a good relationship with a child and for religious reasons disown him or her at disclosure; the parent who "accepts" his or her child's sexual orientation but refuses to acknowledge the child's partner. These, and many others, are situations that are distinctively related to a gay or lesbian person's life situation. In addition, the cumulative effects of hiding one's identity, the adaptation against which many lesbians and gay men struggle, causes severe stress and dysfunction, which may lead to serious coping complications manifested as a poor fit within the family of origin.

Although much of the available anecdotal evidence has often portrayed the families of gays and lesbians as uncaring and cold-hearted individuals, who immediately disown their family member, once individuals disclose their gay or lesbian identity to them or once they are "found out", this characterization should not be misconstrued as ipso facto in every case. Sources, especially those that are written by parents of lesbians and gay men (Borhek, 1979, 1983, 1988; Dew, 1994; Fairchild and Hayward, 1989; Griffin, Wirth, and Wirth, 1986; Parents and Friends of Lesbians and Gays, 1990), address parental reactions to their child's disclosure from a more balanced perspective and may be useful in work with both the gay and lesbian individual and their families. Practitioners should familiarize themselves with the work of Berzon (1992), Brown (1988), Browning (1987), and Shernoff (1984)—all of whom have made significant contributions that have addressed some of the salient clinical issues for gay and lesbian people and their families. Social workers who come in contact with gay men and lesbians need to remember that all people must be viewed within the context of their own families of origin. An ecomap, originally developed by Meyer (1976) and developed by Hartman (1978), or a genogram

(McGoldrick and Gerson, 1985) might be a useful strategy to depict graphically the nature of transactions between families and their environments at a given time within a given context. Family sculpting, the physical positioning of family members of the client' identified family (Shernoff, 1984) in ways that show the family members' perceptions of the dynamics that are present, can help to clarify clients' perceptions of family dynamics and can be an effective means for clients and family members to find alternative ways of dealing with problems in living. Although traditional approaches to family therapy may be adapted to meet the unique needs of gay men and lesbians, a variety of approaches have demonstrated usefulness. Structural approaches (Aponte and Van Deusen, 1981; Lappin, 1988) to family work pioneered by Minuchin (1974), practice from a Bowenian perspective (Bowen, 1971), problem-solving approaches (Compton and Gallaway, 1994; Haley, 1978, 1987), and integrative approaches (Nichols, 1996) are all methods that have been effective and adaptable to working with gay men and lesbians within the context of their families of origin.

The following are some guidelines adapted from previous works (Berzon, 1992; Mallon, in press b; Rothberg and Weinstein, 1996; Shernoff, 1984; Silverstein, 1977) published for practitioners who are assisting gay and lesbian persons within the family context:

1. The first place to start is to ask the family member about issues of sexual orientation. It is important to note in the initial assessment process if there are any other family members who are openly lesbian or gay (an aunt, an uncle, a cousin).
2. The practitioner should also explore how open or how closed the family system has generally been to new ideas and new people.
3. The practitioner should also ask how the family system has dealt with new and unexpected information historically. Such questions can provide insight into the family's flexibility and may assist in determining which family members will be supportive and which will not be.
4. The practitioner should ask the client a series of questions such as Who do they feel most close to?; Who have they confided in and who has confided in them?; Who do they per-

ceive to be the most liberal members of the family and who will handle this information best?; and How does the family grapevine work? Such exploration might help the individual to decide who might be the most supportive family member to disclose to initially, if they choose to disclose. Rothberg and Weinstein (1996) and Shernoff (1984) both recommend the use of genograms and ecomaps as useful tools in this process, helping the individual to graphically depict family systems. These tools allow for matter-of-fact questioning, which can assist in gathering sensitive information.

5. Practitioners should be available to role-play the disclosure process and other family-focused issues with clients. They should explore with the client several perspectives and offer feedback and suggestions on how the transaction can be accomplished more smoothly.

6. Practitioners should help clients to see that coming out to family members is not a one-time situation, but a process. As individuals and their families disclose on a continuum, clients should be encouraged to consider first disclosing to a family member with whom they are emotionally closest.

7. Practitioners should assist clients in developing a plan for orchestrating the disclosure to the family.

8. Practitioners should recommend that clients never disclose to family members when they are in a crisis or in need of emotional support from family (e.g., after a break up).

9. Practitioners should be available to support and meet with parents and other family members. Shernoff (1984) notes that at the outset, this situation usually requires crisis-intervention strategies. At the point of being "found out" or the points at which the young person comes out, parents themselves are usually so needy for emotional support that they might be unavailable to parent the young person. Therefore, the time immediately following the confirmation that their child is gay or lesbian is when they require the greatest amount of nurturance and support from both their child and the practitioner. Siblings will also need assistance during this time and should not be neglected in the process. Encouraging them to explore feelings, providing them with educational

information, and making them aware of support groups for families such as PFLAG (Parents and Friends of Lesbians and Gays) are important parts of this process. Assigning family members readings—bibliotherapy—that can educate and inform them about a wide variety of issues pertaining to lesbians and gay men is also a useful strategy.

10. Practitioners should remain available to assist both the family and the individual in negotiating this process.

CREATING FAMILIES

Although gay and lesbian persons have not always found acceptance within their own families of origin, many have adapted by creating their own nurturing and loving families. Gay men and lesbians have created their own family systems primarily through two means that will be discussed in this chapter: (1) families where gay men and lesbians as single individuals or couples have decided to parent children or (2) families where lesbians and gay men share their lives with other gay men, lesbian, or heterosexually oriented nonrelatives to develop a support network of nonrelated persons that acts as a family of creation.

Families of Creation Among Gay and Lesbian Persons

Although traditionally the basis of family ties among household members is usually consanguinity, it is not unusual for gay men and lesbians to embrace "fictive kin"—close friends, usually nonrelatives, who achieve status as family members (See Dorrell, 1990; Preston, 1995a).[1] Longres (1995, p. 234) notes that the literature which focuses on people-of-color families suggests that ethnic minority families are more involved with extended kin networks than are families from the dominant culture. This phenomenon, most clearly evidenced within Latino family systems, where friends and nonrelatives are embraced as kin (called *compradrazo*), also exists within the gay and lesbian communities.

---

1. Gay men and lesbian women who form couple relationships may also view themselves as family, but these issues are covered more extensively in the chapters by Barranti and McVinney in this text.

The emergence of such family systems within gay and lesbian communities is not primarily cultivated in response to poor economic conditions, as they frequently are in poor Latino communities, but instead, they are generated as an adaptative response. In some cases, though not all, this adaptation is due to a poor person:environment fit between the gay or lesbian individual person and his or her family of origin. However, another much-overlooked example of a family of creation is the gay or lesbian adult child who takes an elderly dependent parent into his or her home when the parent is no longer able to live independently, as characterized by this case:

> Paul and Louis were a committed couple who had lived together for ten years. Both men were steadily employed and lived very comfortably in a three-bedroom condo that they had purchased three years previously. When Paul's diabetic, wheelchair-bound mother could no longer live independently, the couple decided to bring her to their three-bedroom apartment to live with them. Paul had always had a good relationship with his mother, and Louis' parents already lived close by in a neighboring condo. The event that precipitated the formation of this family of creation was the unplanned disability of Paul's mother. Paul's siblings, who had the competing demands of children and less financial resources, were very supportive and indeed relieved by their mother's decision to live with Paul and his partner. Although the creation of this "family" added some stress to the couple's relationship, the fact that Louis' parents had lived near them had prepared them for both the strains and benefits that come with caring for an elderly parent.

Although some families of creation provide those gay men and lesbians who are a part of them with opportunities to receive the familial nutriments from one another that they oftentimes lacked from their biological family systems, in other cases, families of creation also consist of the biological family members as illustrated above.

The isolation of growing up gay or lesbian in a small town or an isolated geographic area of the country compels many gay and lesbian persons to migrate from small suburban and rural communities to larger cities where there are typically larger numbers of gay and lesbian persons. Urban areas usually offer greater opportunities to meet other gay and lesbian persons through involvement in community centers, gay and lesbian organizations, churches, and other social activities.

Migrating to such niches can provide gay and lesbian persons with sanctuary from the effects of oppression and social pollution, but may not mitigate the effects of loneliness and isolation that many people experience when they live apart from their families. As an adaptation, some gay and lesbian persons might opt to become involved in an intimate, coupled relationship, others many choose to live with friends, former partners, and other nonrelatives, thus creating their own family network.

Family of creation serves many important functions for those who are its members: there is generally a focus on intergenerational ties, providing members with opportunities to interact with both elders and children; opportunities to belong to and to be a part of a nurturing unit that is larger than the individual or a couple; and opportunities to be a part of traditions and rituals that are generally accepted as a component of family life. The creation of kinship families of choice fulfills the need for sustenance and nurturing that all individuals require by providing emotional support and social network functions for its members.

Coming together in families of creation groups can help to soothe the stress of dealing with daily societal heterocentrism. The common process of coming out, shared by both gay men and lesbians, which is a psychically draining and multilayered event, bonds gay men and lesbians together in a way that is akin to making us feel as though we are, as Paul Monette once said, "members of a tribe" (Monette, 1993, p. E17). As Weston (1991, p. 106) points out, "Although the category 'fictive kin' has fallen from grace in the social sciences, it retains intuitive validity for many people in the United States when applied to chosen families."

As characterized by the situation described previously, families of creation may experience stress similar to that which is experienced by families of origin. Many families of creation need assistance in healing past relationships and/or in developing new relationships, achieving their goals, and enhancing their well-being. The following vignette demonstrates many of the issues that families of creation may bring into a treatment forum:

> Barbara and Jean and Mike and Javier have been close, close friends for more than ten years. They live in the same apartment building in New York City. Barbara and Jean have been partners for more than eleven years. Mike and Javier have been lovers for fifteen. Barbara is an only child, and her parents are deceased; Jean is estranged from her family because they cannot deal with the fact that she is a lesbian; Mike has a close relationship with his family, but they live on the West coast, and Javier's family lives in the Dominican Republic and do not know that he is gay.
>
> Barbara and Jean and Mike and Javier spend all of their holidays together. They rent a house on Cape Cod together every summer, and consider themselves to be a family. They are a close knit family, they care for one another, they know each other very well. They are there for each other. Three years ago, Jean was diagnosed with breast cancer. During the last year, Jean has become progressively more ill and recently was hospitalized. Jean's illness has been stressful for this family. She has been hospitalized three times in the past three years and visibly suffered through her chemotherapy treatment. Although the greater part of Jean's caretaking is managed by her partner Barbara, all of the members of this family have shared in caring for their family member. Everyone in this family has been affected by Jean's illness.

Dealing with family members who experience chronic illness is a very stressful event in the lives of the family collective (Mailick, 1980). Although the members of the family in the illustration above seem to have made a positive adaptation to their family member's illness, they will need support, opportunities to vent feelings of anger, loss, and grief, as well as opportunities to take a break from managing the ill family member's care. Hospital visiting, which in and of itself can be stressful, can be made more stressful by policies that restrict visiting, in some cases, to family members only. Members of families of creation groups may have difficulty being accepted as family. Members of this particular family unit will need education about their family member's illness, possibly be given referrals to support groups for families dealing with breast cancer, and possibly be given assistance in rebalancing the family system within the context of chronic illness. In essence, this family will need to have available to it all of the resources that any other family unit would require.

The devastating losses incurred by gay and lesbian communities as a result of the crushing effects of the AIDS pandemic have also had serious consequences for those individuals that are members of families of creation. The reflections of one man who was seen for bereavement counseling are representative of many of those who have endured such losses:

> I have had more than eighty friends die of AIDS. I probably have had more, but I just stopped counting at eighty. Everyone who I have been close to in the past ten years is now dead. I mean these are people whom I spent every Christmas with, people who were my support system, people who were my family. Do you know what that's like? It's like being the only survivor in your family after a terrible catastrophe. It's really hard. It really hurts.

Social workers must be prepared to acknowledge the devastation that AIDS has wrought on these families (See Preston, 1995b; Kantrowitz, 1995). Treating families of creation as legitimate family systems and understanding the importance of these family units in the lives of gay men and lesbians is an essential factor for social workers who are working with gay and lesbian clients. The same theories, frameworks, and methods that are utilized by practitioners with families of origin may also prove useful in working with families of creation.

Gay Men and Lesbians Choosing to be Parents

Gay men and lesbians have always been parents, but until relatively recently, most of these parents had children from heterosexual unions, usually marriage. Although accurate figures are not available, Patterson (1992) estimates that there are between two and eight million gay or lesbian parents in the United States and appraises the number of children of gay or lesbian parents to range from four million to fourteen million. Gay men and lesbians choosing to be parents are apparently increasing numbers (Patterson, 1994, 1995; Weston, 1991).

Gay or lesbian parents may be single, or they may be involved in same-gendered partnerships. Consider the following variations in the structure of gay men and lesbian family life:

1. Gay men and lesbians with children who were born in the context of heterosexual relationships between biological parents, and whose parent or parents subsequently identified as gay or lesbian
2. Gay men who choose to be parents either through adoption, foster care, or surrogacy arrangements
3. Lesbians who choose to be parents through adoption, foster care, or biological birth
4. Lesbians and gay men who choose to coparent with one another through biological means
5. Same-gendered couples and a former spouse (either heterosexual or gay or lesbian) and children from prior unions, constituting a blended family

Parenting in a society that presumes heterosexuality poses many challenges to gay men and lesbians regardless of the family configuration. Many of the issues that social workers may encounter in practice with lesbians and gay men who create families through parenting are very similar to issues faced by heterosexually oriented couples or individuals: concerns about one's ability to parent; concerns about how children will affect couple relationships; parental stress; economic concerns about supporting children; stepparenting when a new primary relationship begins, and dealing with issues of discipline and behavior. Other issues are best understood juxtaposed against a backdrop of heterocentrism (Raymond, 1992). Gay and lesbian persons may experience systemic antigay and lesbian discrimination from health care providers, from teachers and school administrators, from employers, and from those within the legal system (Hunter and Polikoff, 1976). Gay men and lesbians must also contend with many issues that have to do with gender role strain. Two men choosing to parent together or two women choosing to be mothers as a couple must negotiate and work together to decide who does what with respect to parenting. For gay men and lesbians choosing to create families (Martin, 1993), these roles have not been as clearly differentiated by society as they have for heterosexually oriented couples who parent.

Although there has recently been a flood of literature about gay and lesbian parenting (Benkov, 1994; Bigner, 1996; Bozett, 1987; Martin, 1993; Muzio, 1993, 1996; Pies, 1985; Rothman, 1996), the reality of gay men and lesbians as a family rearing children is still an idea that is shocking to many (Roberston, 1996; Vaughan, 1996). The myth of gay men and lesbians as child molesters (Groth, 1978; Newton, 1978) is so powerfully ingrained in the psyche of most people in Western society that the idea that they would be parents seems to be almost unbelievable. The fact is, however, that sexual orientation has nothing to do with one's ability to parent (Child Welfare League of America, 1995). Furthermore, the desire to parent is not exclusively the domain of those individuals who are heterosexually oriented, but is a powerful desire of many men and women who are gay and lesbian (Iasenza, 1996; Shernoff, 1996).

Although the literature on lesbians choosing to parent is plentiful (Mitchell, 1996; Patterson, 1996; Pies, 1985; Riley, 1988), the literature on gay men choosing to be parents is sparse (Frommer, 1996; McPherson, 1993; Sbordone, 1993; Shernoff, 1996). Consequently, this section deals with family issues that are unique to gay fathers. Many of these issues are related to the gender role strain inherent in having two parents of the same gender. Although Western society has within recent decades reconfigured the gender-bound roles of males and females that existed in families during the 1950s and 1960s, mothers are still expected to play a much larger role in child rearing than are fathers. Anyone who doubts this need only to watch television for one hour to see how many commercials focus on children and their dads. Because most men in Western society are not socialized to parent and to nurture children, and instead are socialized to succeed at work and to find their fulfillment in life through accomplishments in the workplace, two men who choose to parent together must learn to negotiate each and every role that they face together as parents. Negotiating roles within an environment that does not generally acknowledge the existence of gay men as parents can be stressful, but it can also have some important benefits.

Although gay fathers may seek social work intervention for a number of reasons that other men may seek assistance, the following case example highlights the several areas that might be the focus of attention:

> John, age thirty-four, and Mark, age forty, have lived together as a couple in a committed relationship for eight years. John is Caucasian. Mark is Latino. They own a home in a suburb of a large metropolitan city in the Southern part of the United States. John owns his own printing business. Mark is a social worker. Over the years, both men have discussed the possibility of parenting; Mark is more enthusiastic about the idea than John, but both have always wanted to have their own family. After reading April Martin's (1993) book *The Lesbian and Gay Parenting Handbook,* and debating all of the options of parenting that are open to them, the men decide on adoption rather than foster parenting, coparenting, or surrogacy. Since Mark is a social worker and knows of the various child welfare agencies within their community, it is Mark who takes the initiative to contact a local child welfare agency to begin to discuss the possibility of adoption. After a great deal of discussion, Mark and John decide to present themselves as an openly gay couple rather than trying to hide the fact that they were gay and to adopt as a single person. Since their city has a nondiscrimination clause based on sexual orientation, they believe that they will be given a fair chance at adopting a child.
>
> As part of the process, they are told that they will have to attend six classes concerning the adoption process and becoming a parent, and will ned to complete a lengthy application form, obtain three references from people who can vouch for their reputations and attest to their ability to parent, give complete financial disclosure statements, submit to a physical exam, and participate in a series of visits to their home and interviews with them (called a home study process). These are conditions that all persons who are interested in adoption must

follow. John and Mark agree to all of these conditions and complete all of the interviews and necessary paperwork in a timely fashion.

During the course of this process, Mark and John are challenged by the social worker, who seems to be fairly well versed on how to work with gay people, to look at their reasons for wanting to parent and to look at how parenting will change their lives. The social worker also informs them that only one of the men could be the legal parent and therefore be listed on the adoption papers. The men decide that since Mark was the one who was most enthusiastic that he should be the legal parent. They agree that John will be the legal guardian and plan to meet with their attorney to make these arrangements. After the home study is completed, the agency identifies for them a three-week-old Latina girl who was born cocaine dependent. They decide to accept this child with love into their home and to start their family life together. The baby is named Margarita.

Both partners are anxious as they are learning to be parents: changing diapers, taking turns getting up for feedings, and spending time with her is all new for them. Mark had decided prior to Margarita's arrival that he would take a family leave from his job. John continues to manage his business. Within two weeks, however, the stress of caring for an infant begins to manifest itself on the couple. John's family, who lives nearby, have remained uninvolved and have not been very supportive about their decision to adopt. Mark's family has been somewhat more supportive, and his mom has come over several times to help out. Many of their gay male friends were initially unsupportive about their decision to adopt, but several have since reconsidered and are very happy to be "uncles" for Margarita.

As Mark stays home to care for Margarita, John goes to his office. When John comes home from work, Mark, who has traditionally cooked their meals, has often not had time to prepare a meal for them. Mark complains of being fatigued from caring for Margarita and is often sleep deprived as the baby does not yet sleep through the night. John feels left out many times, as it is obvious to him that Mark has a deeper bond with Margarita than does he. John begins to resent the time that it takes to parent and wonders if maybe it was a mistake to not have insisted that he be recognized as the legal parent. Both men had no idea how much time it would take to adjust to their new roles as parents, and with limited support from family and friends, they frequently feel isolated and alone. They have heard that there are groups for gay and lesbian parents, but neither of them has had the time to check them out before the baby came, and the nearest group is more than 125 miles away.

Clearly, these men are dealing with several issues that are common for gay men choosing to be parents. Although many of the stresses illustrated above have more to do with first-time parenting issues than with gay dads parenting, there are some unique features to this case example. Unlike their heterosexual counterparts, who couple, get pregnant, and give birth, gay and lesbian individuals and couples who wish to parent must consider many other variables in deciding on whether or not to become parents. First the couple must decide how they should go about creating a family—through adoption (Colberg, 1996), foster parenting (Ricketts, 1991; Ricketts and Achtenberg, 1990), surrogacy, or alternative insemination. Second, the couple must decide whether or not to be open about their sexual orientation. Although it is legal for gay men and lesbians to adopt, (New Hampshire and Florida do ban gay men and lesbians from adopting), some couples, fearing that they would not be able to adopt if they disclosed their orientation, opt for silence. Others choose to be open, and still others identify as "friends" who will raise the child together. Since only one of the same-gendered couple can legally adopt, one of the most significant factors that must be discussed is who will be the legal parent. Since only one parent can be recognized as the legal parent, this establishes, as Hartman (1996, p. 81) points out "an asymmetrical relationship between the two parents and the child, a asymmetry that the parents face on a regular basis as they deal with everything from school visits, medical permission forms, to eligibility for Social Security survivors' benefits in the case of the death of a co-parent, lack of support from biological family that would have been present for most heterosexual couples who parent, to requirements for support and visiting arrangements in the case of a separation."

In the case outlined above, although Mark and John were diligent in working toward adopting a child and moved through the process of the home study and the seminars with ease, like many parents, they had no idea how much of a change a baby would make in their lives. The perceived lack of family support and even support from friends within the gay or lesbian communities, which is a fairly common story heard from gay men and lesbians choosing to be parents, has made the adjustment of this new family all the more difficult. Add to this the fact that their relationship as a couple has been transformed from a duo into a trio with one of the members requiring almost constant attention and factor in a complete shift in the roles that they were comfortable in as a couple, and it is not difficult to see why this is a family that might need some social work intervention. This family could have been greatly assisted by participating in a group for gay men and lesbians who are parents. The presence of a supportive network of other gay or lesbian parents could also have assisted greatly in helping this family make a smoother transition, but ongoing discussions about the changing nature of their relationship as a couple are also a necessary ingredient for success.

As this family's identity as a family became more settled, the couple began to feel more comfortable in their new roles. In the years to come, as this family grows, the men will be continually challenged to develop their identities as gay fathers. These dads will have to deal with the stress of strangers asking questions such as: "Where's her mother?" and "Are you two men raising this little girl all by yourselves? Don't you think she needs a mother figure?" They will also have to deal with the societal bias that perceives of men as individuals incapable of parenting small children.

John and Mark will also have to deal with how to handle disclosing their orientation to their child, as well as how to negotiate with health care professionals, teachers, neighbors, parents of their child's friends, and others within community and organizational settings.

Geography also plays a role in this process; in general, gay men and lesbians who are parents are more likely to find acceptance in urban areas than in rural or suburban ones. Social workers who work with gay fathers must be sensitive to the issues that confront men who deal on a daily basis with an identity that is by and large incongruous to what society believes that men and fathers should be.

Lesbians who choose to parent may also have difficulties that may have less to do with societal expectations of women who parent and more to do with perceptions that heterosexual culture is generally not accepting of lesbian lives (Albro and Tully, 1979; Chafetz, Sampson, Beck, and West, 1974; Hall, 1978; Jones, 1978; Levy, 1992; Lewis, 1980; Lewis, 1984; Loewenstein, 1980; Muzio, 1996). Gay and lesbian individuals who choose to adopt as a single parent will also face stresses that are probably more unique to single parenting, but will also encounter stresses that are specific to being a single gay or lesbian parent, including dating and finding a potential spouse within the nonchild-centered gay and lesbian community.

Lesbian mothers and gay dads often live in fear that they will lose their children. This fear has a real basis in truth, as it is legal in four states—Virginia, Arkansas, Missouri, and North Dakota—for courts to remove custody from lesbian mothers based on the grounds that living with a same-gendered partner makes them unfit mothers (Longres, 1995, p. 250). These fears create stress that can erode and break the bond that keeps a family system together. Without a doubt, having a child changes the dynamic of a relationship or an individual's life, adds stress, and in some cases forces couples who may not have been open about their identity to more openly identify as lesbian or gay, but there are also many benefits to gay and lesbian parenting that far outweigh the drawbacks. Gay men and lesbians who choose to create families have the advantage of redefining and reinventing their own meaning for family and parenting precisely because they exist outside of the traditionally defined family and parenting roles based on gender (Benkov, 1994). In creating their own families, gay men and lesbians offer their own uniqueness and gifts to the children whom they rear and to the larger society's concept of the family and parenting experience.

CONCLUSION

There is no question that many families undergo a transformational process when they learn that a family member is gay or lesbian or when gay or lesbian family members decide to create family networks of their own. The question is if the change will make the family system stronger and draw its members into a closer and more honest relationship, or if the disclosure or creation will generate the sort of conflict that destroys the system and marks its members for the rest of their lives. In discussing the ecosystemic approach to working with clients, Meyer (1988, p. 280) notes, "Systems survive when they maintain equilibrium . . . changing within tolerable limits, and theoretically regenerating themselves to move on to a higher level of functioning." Families, when faced with a myriad of new events, can usually absorb them, and consequently, when this occurs, life can regain a sense of balance. If, on the alternative side, there are unique features of the individual family members or the collective body that are threatened by these events and resulting in stress, then a "loss of equilibrium can take place and the family may be flooded with influences, energy, information, or experiences which they cannot absorb into their way of living" (Meyer, 1988, p. 280). The family's imbalance, as evidenced in each of the case studies presented in this paper, could lead to a chronic state of crisis; however, the same imbalance, and the stress that it creates, could also produce a change within the family system.

In the case of practice with gay men and lesbians within the context of family, maintaining or realigning the balance of the family system is a major treatment goal, but as Meyer (1988, p. 281) points out, "The paths to that end are multiple."

Since many families of origin view disclosure or "discovery" as an intense familial crisis, families will need support, encouragement, and accurate information during and after a family member's disclosure of gay or lesbian orientation. Without appropriate supportive interventions, a family member's disclosure of homosexuality may lead to a complete deterioration of the family system (Savin-Williams, 1989; Strommen, 1989). Practitioners who are educated to the stresses and strains that lesbian and gay persons encounter in the larger heterosexual context are in a good position to offer counsel and empathy.

Practitioners must equally be aware of the damaging effects of hiding one's orientation from families (Berger, 1990; Brown, 1991; Cain, 1991a, 1991b; Martin, 1982;). Gay men and lesbians who choose not to come out to their families experience stresses that are unique to their situations. These stresses seem to particularly manifest themselves around the holidays, when many gay men and lesbians visit with their families of origin. Social workers must be prepared to offer support, encouragement, and guidance during these stress-filled times.

When working with families of creation, practitioners must be educated about and sensitized to the need that all people have to be part of a family unit. Gay men and lesbians who choose to parent experience stresses that may have more to do with parenting issues than with being a gay man or lesbian, but also experience role strain and negative reactions from society that very much have to do with their sexual orientation. These families will need knowledgeable and unbiased professionals to assist them in negotiating the stresses of being a part of a family in a society that presumes heterosexuality. Family units formed by creation are also important realities in the lives of many gay men and lesbians and fulfill important nurturing and sustaining functions that help soothe the damaging effects and stresses of living within a hostile environment. Social workers working with families in this situation must be sensitive to the issues of families of creation and need to respect and honor such systems as genuine family units.

In sum, as social workers, we need to be as knowledgeable as possible about gay and lesbian culture and gay and lesbian experiences, not in ways that lead us to make assumptions, but also to be fully present to clients by really listening to them. To ask questions, and then to really listen to the answers in such as way as the answers will inform us and guide us as only local knowledge can guide practice. In doing so we have the opportunity to not only recognize and identify problems that gay men and lesbians face within the context of families, but also to acknowledge and know the strengths and resilience that many gay men and lesbians possess. There is a manifest need in social work for practitioners to listen to the stories of gay men and lesbians themselves, and also to the stories of their families. Practitioners who are aware of and who are able to truly listen and respond with empathy and knowledge are best situated to assist families in remaining intact and in helping them move toward healthfulness.

REFERENCES

Adair, N. and Adair, C. (1978). *Word is out: Stories of some of our lives.* New York: Dell.

Albro, J. and Tully, C. (1979). A study of lesbian lifestyles in the homosexual micro-culture and the heterosexual macro-culture. *Journal of Homosexuality, 4*(4), 331-344.

Allen, K. R. and Demo, D. H. (1995). The families of lesbians and gay men: A new frontier in family research. *Journal of Marriage and the Family, 57,* 1-17.

Aponte, H. and Van Deusen, J., (1981). Structural family therapy. In A. Gurman and D. Knisken (Eds.), *Handbook of family therapy* (pp. 310-360). New York: Brunner/Mazel.

Benkov, L. (1994). *Reinventing the family: The emerging story of lesbian and gay parents.* New York: Crown Publishers.

Berger, R. M. (1982). The unseen minority: Older gays and lesbians. *Social Work, 27*(3), 236-242.

Berger, R. M. (1984). Realities of gay and lesbian aging. *Social Work, 29*(1), 57-62.

Berger, R. M. (1990). Passing: Impact on the quality of same-sex couple relationships. *Social Work, 35*(4), 328-332.

Berzon, B. (1992). Telling your family you're gay. In B. Berzon (Ed.), *Positively gay: New approaches to gay and lesbian life* (pp. 67-78). Berkeley, CA: Celestial Arts.

Bigner, J. (1996). Working with gay fathers. In J. Laird and R-J. Green (Eds.), *Lesbians and gays in couples and families: A handbook for therapists* (pp. 370-403). San Francisco: Jossey-Bass Publishers.

Blumenfeld, W. and Raymond, D. (1988). *Looking at gay and lesbian life.* Boston: Beacon Press.

Borhek, M. V. (1979). *My son Eric.* New York: Pilgrim Press.

Borhek, M. V. (1983). *Coming out to parents.* New York: Pilgrim Press.

Borhek, M. V. (1988). Helping gay and lesbian adolescents and their families: A mother's perspective. *Journal of Adolescent Health Care, 9*(2), 123-128.

Bowen, M. (1971). The use of family theory in clinical practice. In J. Haley (Ed.), *Changing families* (pp. 159-192). New York: Grune and Stratton.

Bozett, F. W. (1987). *Gay and lesbian parents.* New York: Praeger.

Brown, L. (1988). Lesbians, gay men, and their families. Common clinical issues. *Journal of Gay and Lesbian Psychotherapy, 1*(1), 65-77.

Brown, P. (1991). Passing: Differences in our public and private self. *Journal of Multicultural Social Work, 1*(2), 33-50.

Browning, C. (1987). Therapeutic issues and intervention strategies with young adult lesbian clients: A developmental approach. *The Journal of Homosexuality, 13*(4), 45-53.

Cain, R. (1991a). Relational contexts and information management among gay men. *Families in Society, 72*(6), 344-352.

Cain, R. (1991b). Stigma management and gay identity development. *Social Work, 36*(1), 67-73.

Carter, B. and McGoldrick, M. (Eds.). (1989). *The changing family life cycle: A framework for family therapy,* second edition. Boston: Allyn and Bacon.

Chafetz, J. S., Sampson, P., Beck, P., and West, J. (1974). A study of homosexual women. *Social Work, 19*(6), 714-723.

Child Welfare League of America (1995). *Issues in lesbian and gay adoption.* Washington, DC: Child Welfare League of America.

Colberg, M. (1996). With open arms: The emotional journey of lesbian and gay adoption. *In the Family, 2*(1), 6-11.

Compton, B. and Gallaway, B. (1994). *Social work processes,* fifth edition. Belmont, CA: Wadsworth.

Dank, B. M. (1971). Coming out in the gay world. *Psychiatry, 34,* 180-195.

D'Augelli, A. R. and Hershberger, S. L. (1993). Lesbian, gay, and bisexual youth in community settings: Personal challenges and mental health problems, *American Journal of Community Psychology, 21*(4), 421-448.

DeVine, J. L. (1984) A systematic inspection of affectional preference orientation and the family of origin. *Journal of Social Work and Human Sexuality, 2,* 9-17.

Dew, R. F. (1994). *The family heart: A memoir of when our son came out.* Reading, MA: Addison-Wesley.

Dorrell, B. (1990). Being there: A support network of lesbian women. *Journal of Homosexuality, 20*(2/4), 89-98.

Fairchild, B. and Hayward. N. (1989). *Now that you know: What every parent should know about homosexuality.* New York: Harcourt Brace Jovanovich, Publishers.

Frommer, M. S. (1996). The right fit: A gay man's quest for fatherhood. *In the Family, 2*(1), 12-16, 26.

Germain, C. B. (1979). Ecology and social work. In C. B. Germain (Ed.), *Social work practice: people and environments* (pp. 1-22). New York: Columbia University Press.

Germain, C. B. (1991). *Human behavior in the social environment.* New York: Columbia University Press.

Germain, C. and Gitterman, A. (1980). *The life model of social work practice.* New York: Columbia University Press.

Germain, C. and Gitterman, A. (1996). *The life model of social work practice,* second edition. New York: Columbia University Press.

Gilligan, C. (1982). *In a different voice: Psychological theory and women's development.* Cambridge, MA: Harvard University Press.

Griffin, C., Wirth, M. J., and Wirth, A. G. (1986). *Beyond acceptance.* Englewood Cliffs, NJ: Prentice-Hall.

Groth, A. N. (1978). Patterns of sexual assault against children and adolescents. In A. W. Burgess, A. N. Groth, L. L. Holmstrom, and S. M. Sgroi (Eds.), *Sexual assault of children and adolescents* (pp. 3-24). Lexington, MA: Lexington Books.

Haley, J. (1978). *Problem-solving therapy. New strategies for effective family therapy.* San Francisco: Jossey-Bass.

Haley, J. (1987). *Problem-solving therapy. New strategies for effective family therapy,* second edition. San Francisco: Jossey-Bass.

Hall, M. (1978). Lesbian families: Cultural and clinical issues. *Social Work, 23*(5), 380-385.

Hartman, A. (1978). Diagrammatic assessment of family relationships. *Social Casework, 59,* 465-476.

Hartman, A. (1996). Social policy as a context for lesbian and gay families: The political is personal. In J. Laird and R-J. Green (Eds.), *Lesbians and gays in couples and families: A handbook for therapists* (pp. 69-85). San Francisco: Jossey-Bass Publishers.

Hartman, A. and Laird, J. (1983). *Family-centered social work practice.* New York: Free Press.

Hersch, P. (1991). Secret lives. *The Family Therapy Networker, 15* (1), 36-43.

Hess, P. and Jackson, H. (1995). Practice with and on behalf of families. In C. Meyer and M. Mattaini (Eds.), *The foundation of social work practice: A graduate text* (pp. 126-155). Washington, DC: NASW Press.

Hetrick, E. and Martin, A. D. (1987). Developmental issues and their resolution for gay and lesbian adolescents. *Journal of Homosexuality, 13*(4), 25-43.

Hunter, N. D. and Polikoff, N. D. (1976). Custody rights of lesbian mothers: Legal theory and litigation strategy. *Buffalo Law Review, 25,* 691-733.

Iasenza, S. (1996). To have not: The lesbian dilemma. *In the Family, 2*(1), 21-23.

Jones, C. (1978). *Understanding gay relatives and friends.* New York: Seabury Press.

Kantrowitz, A. (1995). Family album. In J. Preston (Ed.), *Friends and lovers: Gay men write about the families they create* (pp. 281-300). New York: Plume.

Kehoe, M. (1988). *Lesbians over 60 speak for themselves.* Binghamton, NY: Harrington Park Press.

Kimmel, D. C. and Sang, B. E. (1995). Lesbians and gay men in midlife. In A. R. D'Augelli and C. J. Patterson (Eds.), *Gay, lesbian, and bisexual identities over the lifespan* (pp. 190-214). Oxford: Oxford University Press.

Laird, J. (1983). Lesbian and gay families. In F. Walsh (Ed.), *Normal family processes,* fourth edition (pp. 282-328). New York: Guilford Press.

Laird, J. (1996). Invisible ties: Lesbians and their families of origin. In J. Laird and R-J. Green (Eds.), *Lesbians and gays in couples and families: A handbook for therapists* (pp. 89-122). San Francisco: Jossey-Bass Publishers.

Lappin, J. (1988). Family therapy: A structural approach. In R. Dorfman (Ed.), *Paradigms of clinical social work* (pp. 220-252). New York: Brunner/Mazel.

Levy, E. F. (1992). Strengthening the coping resources of lesbian families. *Families in Society, 73*(1), 23-31.

Lewis, K. G. (1980). Children of lesbians: Their point of view. *Social Work, 25*(3), 198-203.

Lewis, L. A. (1984). The coming-out process for lesbians: Integrating a stable identity. *Social Work, 29*(5), 464-469.

Loewenstein, S. F. (1980). Understanding lesbian women. *Social Casework, 61*(1), 29-38.

Longres, J. (1995). *Human behavior and the social environment.* Itasca, IL: Peacock.

Lui, P. and Chan, C. S. (1996). Lesbian, gay, and bisexual Asian Americans and their families. In J. Laird and R-J. Green (Eds.), *Lesbians and gays in couples and families: A handbook for therapists* (pp. 137-152). San Francisco: Jossey-Bass Publishers.

Mailick, M. (1980). Impact of serious illness on the individual and family. *Social Work in Health Care, 5*(2), 117-128.

Mallon, G. P. (1992). Gay and no place to go: Assessing the needs of gay and lesbian adolescents in out-of-home care settings. *Child Welfare, 71*(6), 547-556.

Mallon, G. P. (in press a). *We don't exactly get the welcome wagon: The experience of gay and lesbian adolescents in North America's child welfare systems.* New York: Columbia University Press.

Mallon, G. P. (in press b). Gay and lesbian adolescents and their families. In T. DeCrescenzo (Ed.), *Gay and lesbian youth.* New York: Harrington Park Press.

Martin. A. (1993). *The lesbian and gay parenting handbook: Creating and rasing our families.* New York: Harper Perennial.

Martin, A. D. (1982). Learning to hide: The socialization of the gay adolescent. In S. C. Feinstein, J. G. Looney, A. Schartzberg, and A. Sorosky (Eds.), *Adolescent psychiatry: Developmental and clinical studies,* volume 10. Chicago: University of Chicago Press.

McGoldrick, M. and Gerson, R. (1985). *Genograms in family assessment.* New York: Norton.

McPherson, D. (1993). *Gay parenting couples: Parenting arrangements, arrangement satisfaction, and relationship satisfaction.* Unpublished doctoral dissertation, Pacific Graduate School of Psychology.

Meyer, C. (1976). *Social work practice: The changing landscape.* New York: The Free Press.

Meyer, C. (1983). The search for coherence. In C. Meyer (Ed.), *Clinical social work in the eco-systems perspective* (pp. 6-34). New York: Columbia University Press.

Meyer, C. (1988). The eco-systems perspective. In R. Dorfman (Ed.), *Paradigms of clinical social work* (pp. 275-294). New York: Brunner/Mazel.

Meyer, C. (1993). *Assessment in social work practice.* New York: Columbia University Press.

Minuchin, S. (1974). *Families and family therapy.* Cambridge, MA: Harvard University Press.

Mitchell, V. (1996). Two moms: Contribution of the planned lesbian family and the deconstruction of gendered parenting. In J. Laird and R-J. Green (Eds.), *Lesbians and gays in couples and families: A handbook, for therapists* (pp. 343-357). San Francisco: Jossey-Bass Publishers.

Monette, P. (1993 March 15). The politics of silence. *The New York Times*, p. E17.

Muzio, C. (1993). Lesbian co-parenting: On being/being the invisible (m)other. *Smith College Studies in Social Work, 63*(3), 215-229.

Muzio, C. (1996). Lesbians choosing children: Creating families, creating narratives. In J. Laird and R-J. Green (Eds.), *Lesbians and gays in couples and families: A handbook for therapists* (pp. 358-369). San Francisco: Jossey-Bass Publishers.

Newton, D. E. (1978). Homosexual behavior and child molestation: A review of the evidence. *Adolescence, 13,* 205-215.

Nichols, W.C. (1996). *Treating people in families: An integrative framework.* New York: Brunner/Mazel.

Parents and Friends of Lesbians and Gays. (1990). *Why is my child gay?* Washington, DC: Parents and Friends of Lesbians and Gays.

Patterson, C. J. (1992). Children of gay and lesbian parents. *Child Development, 63,* 1025-1042.

Patterson, C. J. (1994). Lesbian and gay couples considering parenthood: An agenda for research, service and advocacy. In L. A. Kurdek (Ed.), *Social services for gay and lesbian couples* (pp. 33-56). Binghamton, NY: Harrington Park Press.

Patterson, C. J. (1995). Lesbian mothers, gay fathers, and their children. In A. R. D'Augelli and C. J. Patterson (Eds.), *Gay, lesbian, and bisexual identities over the lifespan* (pp.262-292). Oxford: Oxford University Press.

Patterson, C. J. (1996). Lesbian mothers and their children: Findings from the Bay area families study. In J. Laird and R-J. Green (Eds.), *Lesbians and gays in couples and families: A handbook for therapists* (pp. 420-438). San Francisco: Jossey-Bass Publishers.

Pies, C. (1985). *Considering parenthood: A workbook for lesbians.* San Francisco: Spinsters/Aunt Lute.

Ponse, B. (1976). Secrecy in the lesbian world. *Urban Life, 5,* 313-339.

Preston, J. (Ed.). (1992). *A member of the family: Gay men write about their families.* New York: Dutton.

Preston, J. (Ed.). (1995a). *Friends and lovers: Gay men write about the families they create.* New York: Plume.

Preston, J. (1995b). Eulogy for George. In J. Preston (Ed.), *Friends and lovers: Gay men write about the families they create* (pp. 83-94). New York: Plume.

Quam, J. K. (Ed.). (1997). *Social services for older gay men and lesbians.* Binghamton, NY: The Haworth Press.

Raymond, D. (1992). "In the best interest of the child:" Thoughts on homophobia and parenting. In W. Blumenfeld (Ed.), *Homophobia: How we all pay the price* (pp. 114-130). Boston, MA: Beacon Press.

Ricketts, W. (1991). *Lesbian and gay men as foster parents.* Portland, MN: National Resource Center for Management and Administration.

Ricketts, W. and Achtenberg, R. (1990). Adoption and foster parenting for lesbians and gay men: Creating new traditions in family. In F. W. Bozett and M. B. Sussman (Eds.), *Homosexuality and family relations* (pp. 83-118). Binghamton, NY: Harrington Park Press.

Roberston, L. (1996 September 3). All clear over surrogate baby. *The Glasgow Herald,* p. 1.

Rothberg, B. and Weinstein, D. L. (1996). A primer on lesbian and gay families. In M. Shernoff (Ed.), *Human services for gay people: Clinical and community practice.* Binghamton, NY: The Haworth Press.

Rothman, B. (1996). Lesbian motherhood—before it was fashionable. *In the Family, 2*(1), 20.

Savin-Williams, R. C. (1989). Parental influences on the self-esteem of gay and lesbian youths: A reflective appraisals models. In G. Herdt (Ed.), *Gay and lesbian youth* (pp.93-110). Binghamton, NY: Harrington Park Press.

Sbordone, A. J. (1993). *Gay men choosing fatherhood.* Unpublished doctoral dissertation. Department of Psychology, City University of New York.

Shernoff, M. (1984). Family therapy for lesbian and gay clients. *Social Work, 29*(4), 393-396.

Shernoff, M. (1996). Gay men choosing to be fathers. In M. Shernoff (Ed.), *Human services for gay people: Clinical and community practice* (pp. 41-54). Binghamton, NY: The Haworth Press.

Silverstein, C. (1977). *A family matter: A parent's guide to homosexuality.* New York: McGraw Hill.

Slater, S. (1995). *The lesbian family life cycle.* New York: The Free Press.

Strommen, E. F. (1989). "You're a what?" Family member reactions to the disclosure of homosexuality. *Journal of Homosexuality, 18*(1/2), 37-58.

Sullivan, T. and Schneider, M. (1987). Development and identity issues in adolescent homosexuality. *Child and Adolescent Social Work, 4*(1), 13-24.

Vaughan, M. (1996 September 3). Dad's out and baby goes too. *The Glasgow Herald,* p. 11.

Weston, K. (1991). *Families we choose: Gay and lesbian kinship.* New York: Columbia University Press.

Chapter 8

Social Work Practice with Lesbian Couples

Chrystal C. Ramirez Barranti

Carmen seemed to be almost glowing today. I had noticed that over the last several sessions she had become increasingly brighter in mood, affect, and expression, a much welcome relief after months of relentless depression. A young woman in her mid-twenties, she had initially come into therapy with questions regarding sexual preference after a breakup of a long-term relationship with a man. I sat expectant as she shifted in her seat, a shifting that often signalled the beginning of our sessions. "I've been wanting to tell you this for a while now," her eyes connecting with mine as I felt her searching for my acknowledgement. "I've met someone," she said. "I've never felt so connected in a relationship before." A long silence followed as her eyes went from searching the carpet to brief contact with me. "Her name is Diane."

This client is embarking on a new journey, not just one of individual self-exploration and identity development, but a journey in experiencing an intimate relationship with a woman. While there has been much said concerning ways in which lesbian couples are dysfunctional, there has been much less said about the positively unique characteristics and dynamics of relationships in which both partners are women.

Special appreciation to Dean Barbara Shank and my colleagues in the School of Social Work at the University of St. Thomas/College of St. Catherine for their dynamic support and encouragement of this work.

Indeed, historical perspectives of homosexuality in general and lesbian couplehood in particular have been pathologically biased (Glassgold and Iasenza, 1995; Green, Bettinger, and Zacks, 1996). For example, from the traditional psychodynamic perspective, homosexuals in general have been viewed as developmentally arrested in the pre-oedipal stage, with consequent primitive psychological functioning and immature object choices (Deutsch, 1995; Lindenbaum, 1985). As a result, lesbians have been described as striving to recreate primal intimacy and merging of the early mother-infant bond in their relationships with other women (Lindenbaum, 1985).

The family therapy field has followed suit in pathologizing perspectives of lesbian couples. For example, the application of family therapy models in work with lesbian couples has traditionally resulted in descriptions of lesbian couples as pathologically fused and enmeshed and consequently made up of undifferentiated adult women (Kreston and Bepko, 1980). Affirming, validating,? Not in the least.

However, the more current research and clinical writing of the past ten years on gender issues, and gay and lesbian individuals and couples have begun to challenge the characteristically pathologizing perspectives of the predominant schools of psychodynamic and family therapy fields (see Glassgold and Iasenza, 1995; Laird and Green, 1996; Roth, 1989; Slater, 1995). This chapter briefly explores the traditional view of lesbian couples as merged, fused, and/or enmeshed in light of the newer and more affirming perspectives that interpret clinical issues of lesbian couples from a broader systems perspective. More specifically, issues related to same-gender socialization, internalized homophobia, and societal oppression and social exclusion are addressed. Common presenting issues brought to therapy by lesbian couples and potential interventions are discussed. Finally, therapist-specific issues in working with lesbian couples are identified.

FUSION AND ENMESHMENT: STRENGTH OR PATHOLOGY?

In all intimate relationships there is a common desire and often consequent struggle to develop a balance between closeness and distance, intimacy and independence, and lesbians couples are no different (Causby, Lockhart, White, and Greene, 1995; Decker, 1984; Roth, 1989). As our client, Carmen, is beginning to realize, one of the most highly valued qualities and strengths of lesbian relationships is the mutual focus on relating to one another that both partners bring to the relationship and the degree of emotional intimacy that follows (McCandlish, 1982; Slater, 1995). While the strength of the lesbian couple can be found in the quality of high emotional connectedness, this has been found to come for some couples at the expense of separateness and individuation (Kreston and Bepko, 1980; McCandlish, 1982; Pearlman, 1989). Given the unique characteristics of lesbian couples, coming to this balance of emotional connection and individuality often comprises a primary focus of the work in couples therapy (Roth, 1989).

Historically, pathological concepts such as merger, fusion, and enmeshment have been used to describe lesbian couples' innate tendency for high emotional closeness as a dysfunction (Deutsch, 1995; Green, Bettinger, and Zacks, 1996; Kreston and Bepko, 1980). More specifically, the concepts of fusion, merger, and enmeshment have been used to describe the loss of individual self and autonomy, as well as the state of undifferentiation of self, which occurs within the relationship as the couple unsuccessfully attempts to balance emotional closeness and individuality (Causby, Lockhart, White, and Greene, 1995; Kreston and Bepko, 1980). A closer examination of fusion and enmeshment is perhaps beneficial as the appropriateness of these concepts for lesbian couples is considered.

Family Therapy Concepts of Fusion and Enmeshment

Fusion and enmeshment, significant concepts in family therapy, have been used to define dysfunctional family relationships that often result in symptomology or dysfunction of one or more family members (Green, Bettinger, and Zacks, 1996). More specifically, the development of individual and relational dysfunction occurs when the individuality and authentic sense of self in relationship are stifled, submerged, or denied in service of maintaining the relationship itself (Bowen, 1978; Green, Bettinger, and Zacks, 1996).

The structural family therapy theory incorporates the concepts of boundaries in gaining understanding of how a family and its subsystems are defined and how they function (Minuchin, 1974). Boundaries of a subsystem are defined by rules which delineate who is included/excluded in the subsystem and how they interact and participate in that subsystem. Providing an identity forming function for systems and subsystems, boundaries are thought to develop along a continuum of emotional closeness ranging from highly diffuse boundaries indicating enmeshment to clear and flexible boundaries indicating healthy adaptation to highly rigid boundaries indicating disengagement (Green et al., 1996). Enmeshment is experienced as intense emotional reactivity, dysfunctional levels of dependency and emotional closeness all occurring at the expense of an individual sense of self and sense of autonomy. Disengagement, on the other hand, involves extreme levels of autonomy and individuality resulting from a lack of emotional reactivity (Minuchin, 1974). According to Minuchin, the couple's task in defining the boundaries of the couple is working out a healthy balance between emotional closeness and individuality within the relational subsystem.

Referring to pathological relational processes, the Bowenian (Bowen, 1978) concept of emotional fusion is expressed through anxiety-driven reactive responses and relational patterns. Since emotional fusion prevents the development and expression of self in service of maintaining the relationship, it stalls the ability for partners to experience themselves as "authentic selves-in-relation" (Green, Bettinger, and Zacks, 1996, p. 187). Triangulation, emotional distancing, unresolved couple conflict, and individual dysfunction are common outcomes of emotional fusion in couple relationships (Bowen, 1978). While attempts at maintaining the relationship, these processes tend to intensify the deferment of self-differentiation and consequently true intimacy (Green, Bettinger, and Zacks, 1996).

While these concepts have been somewhat helpful in understanding and in intervening with troubled lesbian couples, they have been very limiting and perhaps damaging when applied to lesbian couples without a broader perspective of the lesbian couple experience. In fact, unlike with heterosexual couples, the pathological. states of fusion and enmeshment have been used to describe both clinical and nonclinical lesbian couples (Green, Bettinger, and Zacks, 1996). However, recent research has begun to challenge this almost global clinical perception of dysfunction in relation to lesbian couples' innate tendency to high degrees of emotional closeness. For example, some findings have found that while for some couples high levels of fusion become problematic, other couples report high levels of emotional closeness in conjunction with high levels of relationship satisfaction (Causby, Lockhart, White, and Greene, 1995; Green, Bettinger, and Zacks, 1996; Slater, 1995). Understanding when, like in any relationship, quality, coping mechanism, or strength such as emotional closeness is beneficial or becomes problematic is critical for any therapist working with lesbian couples. In developing this understanding or perspective it is helpful to examine the concepts of fusion and enmeshment from a larger perspective that hopefully challenges or reinforms these concepts that have come out of traditional heterosexist and patriarchal perspectives. This is accomplished by exploring the defining characteristics and environmental factors that make lesbian couples unique from heterosexual couples.

In addition to the capacity for desiring and nurturing high emotional closeness, lesbian couples are distinguished from other kinds of couples by several other critical factors: (a) same gender socialization; (b) nonnutritive social environment; (c) internalized homophobia; (d) intersect of sexual identity development and ongoing development of the couple; and (e) issues of sexual intimacy. Since an understanding of the differentiating characteristics and unique challenges of lesbian couples is critical in providing effective therapeutic intervention, exploration of these follows.

INFLUENCE OF SAME-GENDER SOCIALIZATION

The fact that the lesbian couple is comprised of two women may be so obvious that it is also overlooked as a significant factor in defining the relational dynamic of the couple. Chodorow (1978), Gilligan (1982), and others scholars have noted significant differences in female and male development that impact relationship orientation (Berg-Cross, 1988; Miller, 1976). Because of the biological and psychological similarity between mother and daughter, girls develop within an attachment to mother while boys separate. Women then have a developmentally derived preference for emotional closeness, empathy, and mutual sharing in relationships. This capacity for being in relationship is thought by some scholars to support the continual development of a woman's growing identity rather than the squelching of individuality (Miller, 1976; Pearlman, 1989; Slater, 1995). So, when both partners of a relationship are innately oriented toward emotional closeness and the nurturing of relational intimacy, the potential consequence is often a relationship depicted by high emotional connectedness and an experience of sense of self within relationship as opposed to separate from the relationship (McCandlish, 1982; Pearlman, 1989; Peplau, Cochran, Rook, and Padesky, 1978; Roth, 1989).

While same-gender female socialization may be used to explain women's orientation toward and capacity for high emotional intimacy, Pearlman (1989) has noted the potential within female socialization for a maternal expectation of sameness in which individuality and difference are not acceptable. Emotional distancing by mother is often a response to daughter nonconformity such as differing sexual orientation. Women who were socialized within this kind of dynamic may then experience distancing in their primary relationships as indicative of relationship loss. Pearlman (1989, p. 79) goes on to say that a potential consequence of such a developmental experience in adult relationships "is a compulsive responding to the needs and wishes of others and a loss of the primacy of one's own feelings and desires. Ultimately, independence, autonomy, and individuality can become associated with betrayal and loss of others and thus defined as interferences in emotional connectedness." This then may make it difficult for some women to safely develop the flexibility to move away from high levels of emotional connectedness toward more separateness when desired or needed.

THE IMPACT OF A NONNUTRITIVE ENVIRONMENT: HOMOPHOBIA AND SOCIAL EXCLUSION

I had been seeing Charlene and Carol for about ten months. They came into therapy soon after Charlene was diagnosed with breast cancer at age thirty-six. The couple had always thought of themselves as quite self-sufficient. Charlene had been sick now for twelve months. Her cancer had been declared "in remission" only two months ago. Carol was racked with pain at hearing the news that the breast cancer Charlene was so courageously fighting was back with a raging vengeance. Carol wasn't sure what she could do. She was having to rely on friends for help in ways she hadn't ever before. A very private person, she and Charlene had kept a low profile in the community in which they lived as a way to protect their jobs. Working in a poor, rural, southern county school, she didn't dare breathe a word of her intimate relationship with her partner of ten years. How would she ever get through this knowing that she wouldn't be allowed to use her personal leave days to be with just a "friend"? She was acutely distressed, filled with guilt, fear, and shame.

Slater (1995) and others (Decker, 1984; Roth, 1989) have noted that lesbian couples are in fact exposed to persistent and sustaining "lesbian specific" stressors. Such stressors based in homophobia and heterosexism include the lack of social recognition and the lack of social support for the formation and maintenance of the couplehood. In other words, lesbian couples face the challenge of forming a relational system within a social environment that is hostile, invalidating, and excluding. Since a significant component for healthy boundary creation and maintenance is a supportive environment, it is not surprising then that the lesbian couple may form a subsystem characterized by high emotional closeness, and under high degrees of social oppression, a subsystem characterized by enmeshment.

Literally a daily occurrence, the lesbian couple goes into the heterosexist world unrecognized, unmirrored (Buloff and Osterman, 1995). Roth (1989, p. 290) has identified what she calls "bond-invalidating activities," such as the lack of social/legal structures or ceremonies for such bond-sustaining processes as transitioning from dating to a committed partnership; both partners adopting a child together; a partner using the family leave act; partners providing health, retirement, Social Security benefits for one another; and the list goes on. More intimately invalidating perhaps are those actions that occur on the interpersonal level, such as the exclusion of one's partner from family of origin celebrations and gatherings and/or work-related activities and social events.

As one might conclude, the problem of social isolation or lack of affirming social networks can be significant for many lesbian couples and can be highly influential in terms of how a couple forms and maintains its boundaries and creates high emotional closeness or fusion. Unlike the assumed affirming social supports and built-in family of origin supports for heterosexual couples, lesbian couples are left to create their own. "Families of choice" (Weston, 1991) are typically formed by lesbian couples to create their own social support network. Functioning very much like an extended family, "families of choice" are often made up of a tapestry of lifelong friends as well as affirming family members (Green, Bettinger, and Zacks, 1996). Issues related to availability of lesbian communities, severity of external homophobia, shape of internalized homophobia, and issues of sexual identity development and coming out processes for the couple have significant influences on the couple's ability to form and participate in affirming social networks.

Social exclusion or social invisibility is only one element of the homophobic environment. While lesbian couples are challenged with creating defining boundaries of their relationship within a vacuum, they are also challenged with the potential risks of disclosure and visibility (Slater, 1995). Negotiating a social environment that simultaneously denies one's existence while being punishing of visibility is a daily occurrence. Lesbians often must think through whether or not to use the word "we," "I," "us," or "me" when involved in a myriad of social transactions and contexts. Although a moment-to-moment wear on the individuals and couple, the weight of having to negotiate "two worlds" is devastatingly obvious when the couple is in distress or experiencing a painful psychosocial stressor.

INTERNALIZED HOMOPHOBIA

Internalized homophobia is but another impact that the nonnutritive environment has on lesbian couples. Perhaps this is the most hurtful way that this stressor effects partners and the couplehood because it can and often does operate and influence unconsciously. Self-disdain and even self-hatred, low self-esteem, and shame are consequences of internalized homophobia that impacts a partner's experience of self and how she functions in her primary relationship and in the world at large (Buloff and Osterman, 1995; Gair, 1995).

> Internalized homophobia includes unexplored and unresolved feelings of shame in relation to one's sexuality. Shame interferes with recognition, verbalization, and exploration of related feelings, such as intimacy, and contributes to feelings of self-hatred. Internalized homophobia takes something life-affirming, sexuality, and makes it bad. (Gair, 1995, pp. 110-111)

Internalized homophobia finds its way into the experience of the couple. It can easily express as underlying doubt in the viability of the relationship. And, in times of stress, it can be found in the gnawing fear that the relationship cannot weather the conflict or challenges that come up (Slater, 1995).

> Joyce came in to therapy initially stating that she found herself becoming increasingly depressed. She and her partner had been together for seventeen years, having met when they were in their early twenties. Joyce had recently given up a valued teaching position to support her partner's career move to another state. As she mouthed the words, "I want this so much for Lisa, to have her professorship," tears welled up and she collapsed into deep sobs. Realizing that she could not honestly make such a sacrifice for her partner and the relationship, she found herself thinking that this signaled the end, something she didn't want. In fact, valued confidants reflected the same conclusion.

LESBIAN IDENTITY DEVELOPMENT AND COUPLEHOOD

An additional impact of our homophobic society can be found in the experience of sexual identity development (see Cass, 1979; Chapman and Brannock, 1987; Coleman, 1982 for detailed discussion of developmental stages). The effect of growing up in such a pervasively invalidating social environment creates an often disjointed and delayed working through of this developmental process (Buloff and Osterman, 1995; Roth, 1989). It is not uncommon for members of a lesbian couple to be at different stages in their individual lesbian identity developmental process. In fact, it is quite common for this process to not have begun until after actual involvement in a lesbian relationship (Slater, 1995). As is not the case for heterosexual couples, the lesbian relationship grapples with individual identity developmental issues that are directly tied to defining the very couplehood itself. Anxiety, fear, and conflict can result as partners grapple with the internal as well as relational processes of an identity development that is highly stigmatized (Decker, 1984). Distress for the couple can emerge when partners find themselves at different places in this developmental process (Roth, 1989). For example, Roth and Murphy (1986, as cited in Roth, 1989) have noted that the slower movement of one partner can be experienced by the other as threatening to the relationship, while the faster movement of one partner can be experienced by the other as threatening to her current sense of self and sense of security and safety in a homophobic world (Roth, 1989).

> Marsha sat outraged as she listened to Peggy talk about "de-dyking" the house in preparation for her parents' visit for the holidays. Through tears of rage and hurt, she expressed that she could no longer be a part of the systematic removal of all traces of lesbian-related literature, the photos of their vacations, all indications of their couplehood, including the makeup of a second bedroom. After four years of being together, Marsha began to experience Peggy's closeted presentation to her parents as a deep betrayal of their relationship and rejection of her as her partner. She wanted Peggy to tell her parents.

Often it is the intersection of individual identity development issues and the related coming-out processes with the ongoing development and growth of the couplehood that can create enough distress for the couple to seek therapy (Roth, 1989; Slater, 1995). For example, Slater (1995, p. 27), in her work on the most comprehensive model of five stages of lesbian family life-cycle development to date, notes,

> . . . during transitions between relational life cycle stages, the partners must assess the compatibility not only of what

changes each wants for the relationship, but also of what degree of increased visibility their individual lesbian identities can tolerate . . . the couple may react awkwardly to transitions both in the course of their relationship (which pressure the partners for furthered personal development) and in either partner's development of an individual lesbian identity (which requires accompanying relational change).

Offering a map for lesbian couples, Slater (1995) delineates five stages of the lesbian family life cycle, each of which have unique life cycle tasks, relational transitions, and stage-related issues. Table 8.1 lists these stages and provides examples of some of the related tasks and issues.

SEXUAL INTIMACY ISSUES

One of the areas of complaints for lesbian couples has been that of sexual intimacy. In fact, it has been noted that among both clinical and nonclinical samples alike, lesbian couples' primary complaints about sexual expression have been related to (a) infrequency of genital sex and (b) differential desire for genital contact (Roth, 1989). Comparative research of lesbian, gay, and heterosexual couples evidence that of all of these types of couples lesbian couples reported the lowest frequency of genital sex and the greatest decline of genital contact after the second year of the relationship (Blumstein and Schwartz, 1983). However, despite the dissatisfaction with frequency of genital sex, lesbians continue to report high levels of satisfaction with the qualitative experiencing of their overall sex lives (Blumstein and Schwartz, 1983; Kirkpatrick, 1991; Roth, 1989). Lower frequencies of genital contact do not mean lower frequencies of sexual expression and experiencing for lesbians, however. In fact, lesbians report higher frequencies than gay and heterosexual couples of nongenital physical contact such as hugging, cuddling, touching, and kissing, and consider this to be a complete sexual experience in itself (Blumstein and Schwartz, 1983; Loulan, 1984). If this is the case, how is it that couples often present to therapy for treatment with issues of sexual intimacy? Perhaps some understanding of this dilemma can be found in the

TABLE 8.1. Slater's Five Stages of the Lesbian Family Life Cycle

Stage	Examples of Tasks	Examples of Issues
One: Formation of the Couple	Becoming a unit Healthy conflict management Negotiating visibility as a couple	Building trust Pacing issues of degree of closeness and commitment Difficulty assessing significance of meaning of conflict
Two: Ongoing Couplehood	Increased joining and integration into daily lives Short-term commitment Learning about partner's values, personality, defensive styles Sexual expression and deep emotional bonding Limerance (compatibility) replaced with commitment	Validation of couplehood Influence of past relationships Fears of rejection and abandonment exposed Intense fusion Intimacy issues
Three: The Middle Years	Permanency and long-term commitment Family rituals Belief in partner's ability to grow, change Balance search for newness with stability Reworking of rewards, limitations, and commitment	Fear generated by realization of lifetime with partner's imperfections Experience partner's limitations as stifling to self-growth Feared relational mortality: intensified if in mid-life Inhibited interaction Resistance/denial of conflict Potential for triangulation
Four: Generativity	Developing deeper sense of relational purpose Individual and joint generative efforts Enjoyment of relational maturity and stability May choose parenthood May launch children	Missed opportunities for intimate connection Increased stress if not "out" Impact of midlife physical changes, partner life stages, extended family changes

| Five: Lesbian Couples Over 65 | Adjustment to imposed life changes
Rework balance of separateness and togetherness
Adjustment to health-related changes
Widowhood | Processing of symbolic losses
Fears of loss of autonomy
Sexual intimacy issues
Losses of perceived self-sufficiency due to retirement
Impact of lack of couple-affirming social services |

Note: Not a comprehensive summary. From Slater, S. (1995). *The lesbian family life cycle*. New York: The Free Press.

influences of female socialization and the impact of external and internal homophobia on sexual expression.

Not much is truly known about women's sexuality apart from males. Lesbians, like all women, have been socialized in traditional heterosexist culture in which women are taught to be sexually responsive to someone else and to repress one's own sexual desires. An additional layer of repression of sexual desire occurs for lesbians and bisexual women, who additionally learn from an early age to inhibit their natural sexual desire for another of the same gender because of negative social repercussions of oppression and stigmatization (Loulan, 1984). Internalized homophobia and its consequent self-shame about one's sexuality can play an inhibiting role in sexual desire as well as sexual expression (Gair, 1995).

Differences in partner desire, frequency, and problems related to initiation of sex are commonly identified by lesbian couples (Kirkpatrick, 1991; Loulan, 1984). Unlike heterosexual women, lesbian women may have fewer of the typical opportunities to discuss such issues with typical confidants such as sisters, mothers, etc., and may have difficulty normalizing issues that may be worked out through open communication with one's partner. As Kirkpatrick (1991) has pointed out, however, some couples need therapeutic support and encouragement to voice differences around sexual expression since the very act of expressing differences of any kind may be initially experienced as threatening to the relationship.

Other consequences of a homophobic environment relate to the complete absence of same-sex images in an otherwise highly sexualized culture. Typically, most lesbians live a majority of their waking and working hours in an environment where the automatic reflex is to inhibit displays of physical affection such as holding hands, kissing, and walking arm in arm for fear of very real and negative consequences. This process of chronic situation-specific inhibition may make it more effortful to allow for awareness of sexual desire and expression of sexual behavior when in fact it is safe to do so (Buloff and Osterman, 1995; Pearlman, 1989; Roth, 1989). Sometimes helping the couple to identify the impact that living in two worlds may be having on their sexual awareness and expression can be very freeing.

> Ann and Sophie initially sought therapy for what they de-scribed as general worries about how they were getting along. The couple had been under a considerable degree of stress, having recently relocated and taken on new jobs. They had been living for the past four months with a heterosexual friend and her two preadolescent children while they had a home built. They described their friend as very supportive and also described having to be watchful for any overt displays of verbal or physical affection when outside of their bedroom. After several sessions, Sophie very shyly began to talk about how much she missed Ann, although they were tucked in a one-bedroom living space. As she mustered her courage, she shared that after eight years of an enjoyable and active sex life, they both seemed to becoming increasingly disinterested and then inhibited when the desire was present. They both felt a sense of rejection from one another and identified confusing feelings of shame.

As discussed earlier, the development of extreme emotional closeness has been identified as an attempt at boundary creation and maintenance in a homophobic environment. While resulting issues related to loss of self and individuality occur, further consequences are seen in the area of sexual expression. In fact, genital sexual infrequency among lesbian couples has also been explained as a consequence of prolonged extreme fusion or merger in the relation-ship (Lindenbaum, 1985; Pearlman, 1989). In an attempt to allay the anxiety generated by a sense of loss of self and loss of separate-ness, the couple finds themselves experiencing a gradual decline in sexual activity and potentially a total absence of sex in the relationship (Lindenbaum, 1985).

FUSION AND ENMESHMENT AS FUNCTIONAL AND ADAPTIVE: HIGH EMOTIONAL CLOSENESS

Having recently turned forty, Ellen had come into therapy for what she described as a "gift to myself." Surprisingly, she found herself confronted with existential life questions as she thought about where she had been, where she is now, and where she might be going. Reflecting on her relationship of eighteen years, she described her deep appreciation for her partner, her support, and the "platform," as she described it, which their years together gave her during this time of internal struggle and self-growth.

Mencher's (1990) qualitative research on lesbian couples found that contrary to traditional views of fusion as preventing individuality, the high degree of emotional closeness in her couples sample was experienced as encouraging of individual growth and trust in the relationship. Green and colleague's (1996) comparative research on nonclinical lesbian, gay, and heterosexual couples found that, indeed, lesbian couples were highly emotionally close. In addition, their research revealed that lesbian couples are more emotionally close and more satisfied with their relationships than were either the gay or heterosexual couples. The adaptive function of high emotional closeness provides a sense of security and couple boundary maintenance in a homophobic and excluding social environment (Decker, 1984; Roth, 1989; Slater, 1995). The adaptiveness of fusion, or rather, high emotional closeness, may be more clearly related to the partner's ability to move fluidly along a continuum of higher and lower levels of emotional closeness without experiencing threats to individualility or to the experience of couplehood (McCandlish, 1982; Pearlman, 1989; Roth, 1989; Slater, 1995). Without this flexibility in moving along the emotional closeness continuum, it is probable that enough distress could occur to bring the couple into therapy. And, as we have seen in the above discussion, there is a plethora of influencing factors that persistently and negatively impinge on the developing couple, making the normal challenge of balancing individuality and emotional connection even more difficult.

FUSION AS PATHOLOGY

It is not surprising that lesbians utilize one of their most valued and inherent relationship strengths in adapting to a nonnutritive environment. The strong focus on the relationship and the nurturance of high levels of emotional closeness help to provide boundary creation and maintenance for the lesbian couple (Roth, 1989; Slater, 1995). The lack of goodness of fit, of a nonnutritive environment with its persistent bond-invalidating stressors intersecting with individual partner issues may for some lesbian couples force the creation of rigid boundaries, a closed system, extremely high levels of fusion and the consequent development of painful distress that leads them to therapy (Green, Bettinger, and Zacks, 1996; Roth, 1989).

For example, rigid or extreme fusion at the expense of individuality can result in unresolved couple conflict or triangulation, two of the common outcomes of fusion (Green, Bettinger, and Zacks, 1996; Roth, 1989). Becoming overly sensitive to partner needs at the expense of one's own needs and denial of individual differences can lead to unexpressed feelings, thoughts, and issues intensifying an avoidance of conflict in the relationship (Pearlman, 1989). Prolonged fusion can lead to a sense of loss of self or an experience of false sense of self resulting in resentment and potentially depression (Pearlman, 1989). Indirect distancing behaviors may be initiated through the process of triangulation. An affair, overinvolvement in work or outside projects, a therapist, or having a child are examples of a third party pulled in by a partner in an ineffective attempt at distancing, which leaves the dynamic of extreme fusion unresolved (Green, Bettinger, and Zacks, 1996; Pearlman, 1989; Roth, 1989). Additional attempts at distancing include sexual disinterest, initiation of arguments, intermittent distancing and closeness by one or both partners in the relationship, and extreme dependency (Burch, 1982; Roth, 1989).

It is no doubt that fusion as a pathological state is sometimes experienced by lesbians couples as a painfully distressing relationship process. It is critical for clinicians to realize that high emotional closeness experienced by most lesbian couples is more often an adaptive and valued quality of their relationship constellation and dynamics. Assessing the quality of couple closeness and distinguishing between what may be true fusion and what may be positive high emotional closeness is a significant factor in any work with lesbian couples (Green, Bettinger, and Zacks, 1996).

> Louise and Sarah had been together for ten years. Having described the first several years of their relationship as an experience of near "blissful" intimacy, they had come into therapy as a couple with concerns about the gradual decline of sexual activity and a growing sense of loneliness. Louise in particular presented with issues related to her growing uneasiness with realizing that she did not know who she was anymore, something Sarah was unable to understand. Louise described her increasing awareness of herself as ineffectual in the relationship, unable to identify her own needs and assert her desires for the direction of her life and her relationship. Sarah expressed feelings of rejection and vulnerability and worried that Louise was no longer in love with her. Sarah described Louise as becoming increasingly more angry and overly critical of her, something Sarah indicated had not been present in their relationship before. They both feared that their relationship was coming to end, something neither of them wanted. They were equally distressed and at a loss as to what to do.

THERAPIST-SPECIFIC ISSUES

In addition to working with and being attuned to common treatment issues presented by any type of couple (unresolved developmental issues, dysfunctional family roles, family of origin issues, communication skills, childhood trauma issues, etc.), effective therapy with lesbian couples requires a thorough knowledge and clinical sensitivity to the unique characteristics and strengths as well as the impact of societal stressors, institutional homophobia, and internalized homophobia have on the lesbian couple. If at any time one is reminded of truly working from a person-in-environment perspective it is when working with the lesbian couple. Homophobia and its insidious influences within the therapist office cannot be a discounted possibility/occurrence for lesbian and gay therapists as well as for the most diversity-sensitive heterosexual therapist (for more detailed discussion, see: Burkhe, 1988; DeCrescenzo, 1984; Gelso, Fassinger, Gomez, and Latts, 1995; Greene, 1994; Markowitz, 1991). Sensitivity to and awareness of how homophobia may be operating within oneself as therapist is critical. For example, a heterosexual therapist may need to pay particular attention to her own comfort level with homoerotic feelings; gender role issues; unawareness of the subtleties of oppression and invisibility; potential omissions and influences of unchallenged heterosexist bias; and lingering influences of pathologically oriented theory and training.

Lesbian and gay therapists are not exempt from the call to be vigilant in relations to homophobia in their work with their clients. The already explored and the unexplored effects of internalized homophobia with its consequent internal experiencing of shame must be periodically and perhaps continuously worked on within oneself as a homosexual person who lives within a homophobic social environment. The fact is that unexamined and unrecognized shame and its effects on oneself and one's life can leave the therapist unable to recognize and work with this powerfully painful experience in lesbian clients (Buloff and Osterman, 1995).

The Lesbian Therapist

McCandlish (1982) has noted that the lesbian therapist in particular may encounter particular countertransferential issues in her work with lesbian couples. She states that the lesbian therapist may want to be observant of the following countertransferential tendencies: overidentification with the couple; overinvestment in the treatment outcome; overromanticizing and idealizing the relationship. Indeed, even one's sensitivity to the impact of homophobia and societal oppression on one's clients may lead to overattribution to the social context at the expense of missing intrapsychic pain, developmental issues, or dysfunctional relational dynamics (Roth, 1989).

Affirming function: In the absence of a validating social environment, the lesbian therapist has an additional aspect to her role as therapist in working with lesbian couples.

> Lesbian couples are hungry to be seen, to be admired for their unique qualities, to be appreciated for their accomplishments. These functions, otherwise served by family and community, are less available to most lesbians. The lesbian-affirmative therapist must be called upon to serve as peer, as teacher, as mother, as grandmother, as aunt, as spiritual and financial and legal advisor. Lesbian couples express deep needs to be told their relationship is going through "normal" difficulties, that they are not alone, that there are others who have traversed this path before successfully. (Kasoff et al., 1995, p. 258)

Boundaries. Acknowledgement and acceptance of the responsibility of professional power and privilege is a critical prerequisite to maintaining ethical therapeutic practice (Peterson, 1992). Particular issues related to professional boundaries may require special vigilance from the lesbian therapist who works within the same community in which she lives. The reality of living and working in the typically close and small lesbian communities more often than not means the therapist likely maintains multiple and overlapping roles beyond those identified in her lesbian-affirming therapist role. She may find herself crossing paths with clients at community events, on the athletic field, in the local women's bookstore, or perhaps in her college classroom. Maintaining professional boundaries in one's small community in which overlapping and multiple roles are the norm requires scrupulous observance and protection (Brown, 1988; Woodman, Tully, and Barranti, 1995).

Self-disclosure. Issues of self-disclosure around sexual orientation and pertinent life experiences of the lesbian-affirming therapist may take on special significance in work with lesbian couples. Perhaps the significance of the use of self-disclosure is made more poignant when placed upon the backdrop of lesbian clients' struggle to develop and define self and primary relationships in a nonvalidating and nonnutritive environment. As always is the guide for use of therapist self-disclosure, it should only be used to benefit the client. In work with lesbian clients, self-disclosure of the therapist's lesbian identity at clinically appropriate times in the therapeutic process may in fact be a critical and necessary intervention for the therapy to be an effective and healing process (Gabriel and Monaco, 1995). In fact, given the severity and pervasiveness of external and internalized homophobia, the question may be if true healing can actually occur for the lesbian client if such self-disclosure is omitted from the therapeutic process (Gabriel and Monaco, 1995).

IN SUMMARY:
THERAPEUTIC GOALS AND INTERVENTIONS

In working with lesbian couples concerning issues of balancing high emotional closeness and individuality/separateness, the therapist may wish to consider the following general treatment guidelines while always keeping in mind the defining characteristics and social contexts of each couple. Figure 8.1 offers a summary of significant factors related to individual, couple, and social variables influencing couple formation and function discussed in this chapter. Table 8.2 offers a summary of the therapeutic guidelines for practitioners working with lesbian couples. Of course, it is critical to realize the unique individuality of each couple who presents for treatment. Consideration of more generic couple issues related to family of origin, unresolved developmental issues, communication skill needs, individual life-cycle developmental issues, etc., should always be maintained. When present, the impact of childhood trauma/abuse on partners and the couple relationship should also be addressed.

CONCLUSION

Given the brutal realities of a homophobic social environment and all of its consequences, the fact that a couple composed of two women arrives at your office for help in working on relationship

FIGURE 8.1. Significant individual, couple, and social factors influencing lesbian couple formation, function, growth, and maintenance.

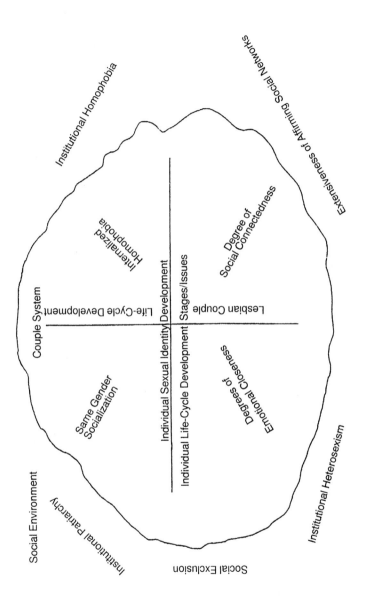

issues at all is a paramount accomplishment. Begin with this realization, consider their positive strengths and qualities, and build on these as together you address the areas of vulnerability and pain. Coming to a balance of connection and individuality is a challenge for all of us, and perhaps a lifelong dance for every lesbian couple. It can truly be a dance of joy and wonderment. It is up to us all.

TABLE 8.2. Therapeutic Guidelines for Working with Lesbian Couples

1. Help the couple to understand and appreciate the impact of homophobia, social exclusion and invisibility, and heterosexism on their experience of themselves as a lesbian couple.
2. Explore the internal experiences of internalized homophobia and its effects on the individual partners as well as on the couple system.
3. Assess individual sexual identity development, coming-out processes and issues, and the potential interface with relationship issues of the couple.
4. Consider life-cycle developmental issues for individual partners and how they may intersect with couplehood issues.
5. Identify lesbian family life-cycle stages and the concurrent issues while considering how these may be interacting with individual identity and developmental issues.
6. Assist the couple in assessing their social support network and promote building an affirming "family of choice."
7. Facilitate each partner's continual development and growth of an individual sense of self within the relationship.
8. Facilitate each partner's ability to tolerate individual differences.
9. Facilitate each partner's ability to tolerate feelings of anger and the experience of conflict and teach healthy anger expression and conflict resolution.
10. Support the experiences of oneself and one's partner as separate by increasing positive tolerance, enjoyment, and acceptance of fluid movement along the continuum of emotional closeness and separateness.
11. Encourage and teach partners to identify their own individual needs and desires as well as how to express them with one another.
12. Address unresolved development issues, family of origin issues, communication skill needs, childhood trauma/abuse if present.
13. Assess issues of sexual expression and assess impact of internalized homophobia, emotional closeness, and socialization, promote communication, and provide education.

REFERENCES

Berg-Cross, L. (1988). Lesbians, family process and individuation. *Journal of College Student Psychotherapy, 3*(1), 97-112.

Blumstein, P. W. and Schwartz, P. (1983). *American couples: Money, work, sex.* New York: William Morrow.

Bowen, M. (1978). *Family therapy in clinical practice.* Northvale, NJ: Aronson.

Brown, L. S. (1988). Beyond thou shalt not: Thinking about ethics in the lesbian therapy community. *Women and Therapy, 8*(1/2), 13-25.

Buloff, B. and Osterman, M. (1995). Queer reflections: Mirroring the lesbian experience of self. In J. M. Glassgold and S. Iasenza (Eds.), *Lesbians and psychoanalysis: Revolutions in theory and practice* (pp. 93-106). New York: The Free Press.

Burch, B. (1982). Psychological merger in lesbian couples: A joint ego psychological and systems approach. *Family Therapy, 9*(3), 201-208.

Burkhe, R. A. (1989). Lesbian related issues in counseling supervision. *Women and Therapy, 8*(1/2), 195-206.

Cass, V. (1979). Homosexual identity formation: A theoretical model. *Journal of Homosexuality, 4,* 219-235.

Causby, V., Lockhart, L., White, B., and Greene, K. (1995). Fusion and conflict in lesbian relationships. In C. T. Tully (Ed.), *Lesbian social services: Research issues* (pp. 67-82). Binghamton, NY: The Haworth Press.

Chapman, B. and Brannock, J. (1987). Proposed model of lesbian identity development: An empirical examination. Journal of *Homosexuality, 14*(3-4), 69-80.

Chodorow, N. (1978). *The reproduction of mothering: Psychoanalysis and the sociology of gender.* Berkeley, CA: University of California Press.

Coleman, E. (1982). Developmental stages of the coming out process. *Journal of Homosexuality, 7*(2-3), 31-43.

Decker, B. (1984). Counseling gay and lesbian couples. In R. Schoenberg, R. S. Goldberg and D. Shore (Eds.), *Homosexuality and Social Work* (pp. 39-52). Binghamton, NY: The Haworth Press.

DeCrescenzo, T. A. (1984). Homophobia: A study of attitudes of mental health professionals toward homosexuality. In R. Schoenberg, R. S. Goldberg, and D. Shore (Eds.), *Homosexuality and social work* (pp. 115-136). Binghamton, NY: The Haworth Press.

Deutsch, L. (1995). Out of the closet and on to the couch: A psychoanalytic exploration of lesbian development. In J. M. Glassgold and S. Iasenza, *Lesbians and psychoanalysis: Revolutions in theory and practice* (pp. 19-37). New York: The Free Press.

Gabriel, M. A. and Monaco, G. W. (1995). Revisiting the questions of self-disclosure: The lesbian therapist's dilemma. In J. M. Glassgold and S. Iasenza, *Lesbians and psychoanalysis: Revolutions in theory and practice* (pp. 161-172). New York: The Free Press.

Gair, S. R. (1995). The false self, shame and the challenge of self-cohesion. In J. M. Glassgold and S. Iasenza (Eds.), *Lesbians and psychoanalysis: Revolutions in theory and practice* (pp. 107-123). New York: The Free Press.

Gelso, C. J., Fassinger, R. E., Gomez, M. J., and Latts, M. G. (1995). Counter-transference reactions to lesbian clients: The role of homophobia, counselor gender, and countertransference management. *Journal of Counseling Psychology, 42*(3), 356-364.

Gilligan, C. (1982). *In a different voice: Psychological theory and women's development.* Cambridge, MA: Harvard University Press.

Glassgold, J. M. and Iasenza, S. (Eds.). (1995). *Lesbians and psychoanalysis: Revolutions in theory and practice.* New York: The Free Press.

Green, R-J., Bettinger, M., and Zacks, E. (1996). Are lesbian couples fused and gay male couples disengaged? In J. Laird and R-J. Green (Eds.), *Lesbians and gays in couples and families: A handbook for therapists* (pp. 185-230). San Francisco: Jossey-Bass.

Greene, B. (1994). Lesbian and gay sexual orientations: Implications for clinical training, practice, and research. In B. Green and G. M. Herek (Eds.), *Lesbian and gay psychology, theory research and clinical applications: Psychological perspectives on lesbian and gay issues: Vol. 1* (pp. 1-24). Thousand Oaks, CA: Sage.

Kasoff, B., Boden, R., De Monteflores, C., Hunt, P., and Wahba, R. (1995). Coming out of the frame: Lesbian feminism and psychoanalytic theory. In J. M. Glassgold and S. Iasenza (Eds.), *Lesbians and psychoanalysis: Revolutions in theory and practice* (pp. 229-264). New York: The Free Press.

Kirkpatrick, M. (1991). Lesbian couples in therapy. *Psychiatric Annals, 8,* 491-496.

Kreston, J. A. and Bepko, C. S. (1980). The problem of fusion in the lesbian relationship. *Family Process, 19,* 277-289.

Laird, J. and Green, R-J. (1996). *Lesbians and gays in couples and families: A handbook for therapists.* San Francisco: Jossey-Bass.

Lindenbaum, J. P. (1985). The shattering of an illusion: The problem of competition in lesbian relationships. *Feminist Studies, 11 (1),* 85-103.

Loulan, J. (1984). *Lesbian sex.* San Francisco: Spinster/Aunt Lute.

Markowitz, L. M. (1991 January-February). Homosexuality: Are we still in the dark? *The Family Therapy Networker,* pp. 26-29, 31-35.

McCandlish, B. M. (1982). Therapeutic issues with lesbian couples. *Journal of Homosexuality, 7*(2), 71-78.

Mencher, J. (1990). Intimacy in lesbian relationships: A critical re-examination of fusion. *Stone Center Working Paper Series, No. 42.* Wellesley, MA: Wellesley College Stone Center for Women's Development.

Miller, J. B. (1976). *Toward a new psychology of women.* Boston: Beacon Press.

Minuchin, S. (1974). *Families and family therapy.* Cambridge, MA: Harvard University Press.

Pearlman, S. F. (1989). Distancing and connectedness: Impact on couple formation in lesbian relationships. *Women and Therapy, 9* (3), 77-88.

Peplau, L. A., Cochran, S., Rook, K., and Padesky, C. (1978). Loving women: Attachment and autonomy in lesbian relationships. *Journal of Social Issues, 34*(3), 7-27.

Peterson, M. R. (1992). *At personal risk: Boundary violations in professional-client relationships.* New York: W. W. Norton.

Roth, S. (1989). Psychotherapy with lesbian couples: Individual issues, female socialization, and the social context. In M. McGoldrick, C. M. Anderson and F. Walsh (Eds.), *Women in families: A framework for family therapy* (pp. 286-307). New York: W. W. Norton and Company, Inc.

Slater, S. (1995). *The lesbian family life cycle.* New York: The Free Press.

Weston, K. (1991). *Families we choose: Lesbians, gays, kinship.* New York: Columbia University Press.

Woodman, N. J., Tully, C. T., and Barranti, C. C. (1995). Research in lesbian communities: Ethical dilemmas. In C. T. Tully (Ed.), *Lesbian social services: Research issues* (pp. 57-66). Binghamton, NY: The Haworth Press.

Chapter 9

Social Work Practice with Gay Male Couples

L. Donald McVinney

Gay male couples are highly diverse. Various social and historical conditions combine with constructs of eroticism, gender, and intimate relationships to create the rich constellations of gay male couples. These include, but are not restricted to, variations of ethnicity, race, class, models of coupling (such as exclusivity verses nonexclusivity, heterosexually married gay men with extramarital gay relationships, and noncohabiting partnerships), longitudinal stage of development, age discrepancies, and cohort of gay identity and coupling formation. Thus, gay male couples must be conceptualized as subcategories within a broader frame of social relations and are not identical to heterosexual couples in structure or form.

Just as it becomes difficult to make unifying statements about gay male couples without stereotyping, generalized descriptions of the difficulties that motivate gay male couples to seek social work services is also problematic. Gay male couples may engage in couples counseling for as many reasons as any other subgroup. However, it may be hypothesized that, similar to their heterosexual counterparts, the majority of gay male couples initiate couples therapy to reduce relational conflict and stabilize the coupling system.

Although tentative, some preliminary remarks can be offered concerning content issues that are expressed by gay male couples requesting social work intervention. These content issues may be influenced by process dynamics inherent in partnerships of two people of the same masculine gender embedded within a nongay culture (Moses and Hawkins, 1986). Common issues of gay male couples involved in couples work may include the following:

1. Conflicts associated with differences in stage levels of being "out" around their gay identity
2. HIV health status concerns
3. Conflicts associated with internalized homophobia
4. Conflicts associated with differences in extended family involvement
5. Conflicts associated with differences in constructions and expectations of coupling
6. Conflicts associated with differences in age
7. Conflicts associated with differences in expectations of sexual exclusivity/nonexclusivity
8. Conflicts associated with perceived inequalities of power and difficulty in negotiating
9. Conflicts associated with chemical use, chemical dependency, and recovery
10. Conflicts associated with finances and financial disparity

An understanding of presenting issues for gay male couples is greatly enhanced by the social worker's attention to interactions of (1) gay male clients' experience of social oppression, (2) issues of male gender role socialization, and (3) the gay male coupling structure. This chapter will address process dynamics and structural variations as they apply to the issues of internalized homophobia, heterosexism, and gay identity development in gay male couples. Through an exploration of these factors, it is hoped that social workers can be assisted in formulating interventions that are specific to gay male couples.

Social work practice with gay male couples is an outgrowth of a family systems perspective (Carl, 1990; Goldenberg and Goldenberg, 1990; Rothberg and Weinstein, 1996). However, family systems theory has limitations. Besides the theoretical tendency to focus on larger systems and less on the two-person system, McGoldrick (1996) notes that most family systems theory and family systems practitioners have traditionally been heterocentric. There is a paucity of attention to gay male couples in the literature, or including gay male couples within the definition of a family, until very recently.

While gay male practitioners with large numbers of gay male clients have always provided services to gay male couples, the emerging literature among family systems theorists has arisen less because of their own spontaneous enlightenment than because of the increasing empowerment of gay male couples. As consumers, gay male couples are demanding equal rights to access mental health services. In their efforts to define the dominant meaning of "family," the radical right and conservative, fundamentalist Christian movement's interjection into national political discourse of definitions of a family in an effort to redefine "traditional family values" has resulted in an oppositional discourse by gay and lesbian families, including gay male couples, who have become more political in advocating for their needs (Hartman, 1996). The increasing insistence that political movements hostile to gay men and lesbians will not define their partnering as anything less than equal to heterosexual couples has become a political issue that has moved increasingly into the legislative arena where at the time of this writing several states in the United States are considering the legal recognition of gay marriages. While this larger political discussion is outside of the parameters of this article, it is helpful for social workers to remember that policy issues impact directly on the lives of the clients we serve and may be the underlying causal factor as to why clients seek services.

Gay male couples can be seen by social work providers in all health and mental health care settings in which there is a social work presence: (1) in hospitals or outpatient clinics, either mainstream (public and private) or health clinics that are gay/lesbian/bisexual/transgender specific; (2) in organizational or industrial settings; (3) in private or independent practice offices; (4) in social services agencies, for instance those serving young people or senior citizens; (5) in HIV/AIDS services organizations; (6) in mainstream or gay/lesbian/bisexual/transgender community centers; (7) in schools and academic settings; (8) in counseling centers; and (9) in chemical dependency treatment programs. While gay male clients are seen in all of the above settings, their sexual identity may remain invisible unless attended to and supported by the social work provider (Rothberg and Weinstein, 1996). Initially, gay men may seek services as individuals and then the gay male partner may be introduced into the practice setting. Gay male couples may also directly present as a couple seeking counseling services. Unfortunately, the assessment of clients' needs may be largely determined by the setting, for instance, residential or community-based; the mission of the agency or institution; the theoretical orientation of the supervisor or department head; or the license under which the agency operates (mental health or substance abuse) rather than client generated. Intervention strategies and outcome goals will largely follow from the initial and ongoing assessment (Meyer, 1993).

INTERNALIZED HOMOPHOBIA, HETEROSEXISM, AND GAY IDENTITY

Although the concepts of internalized homophobia, heterosexism, and gay identity are covered elsewhere in this collection, the redundancy here is intentional as these concepts have particular bearing on and particular significance for the gay male couple. Homophobia can be defined as the irrational fear of gay/lesbian people. Internalized homophobia is defined as "the taking in or internalization of society's negative attitudes and assumptions about homosexuality by gays and lesbians" (Bozett and Sussman, 1990, pp. 337-338). Negative beliefs and attitudes about homosexuality and gay men are naturally absorbed in a heterosexist and homophobic culture by gay and straight people alike. For gay men, however, the effects of this internalization are particularly pernicious (Biery, 1990; Isensee, 1991; Malyon, 1985; Weinberg, 1972). Internalized homophobia has been implicated as the cause for significantly higher rates of chemical dependency in the gay/lesbian community (Finnegan and McNally, 1987), gay/lesbian adolescent suicide (Savin-Williams, 1990), low self-esteem and social isolation, and difficulties in establishing or maintaining intimate relationships among gay men.

Socially constructed negative attitudes and myths about gay men are easily identified and include the following:

1. Most gay men are effeminate.
2. Most gay males in relationships adopt passive/active sexual and gender roles.
3. All gay men are sexually promiscuous.

4. Gay men believe they are women trapped in men's bodies.
5. Most gay men would have a sex change operation if they could.
6. Most gay men are child molesters.
7. Most gay people are miserable, lonely, and psychologically disturbed.
8. Gay relationships never last.
9. Homosexuality is unnatural.
10. Homosexuality affects a minute segment of the population.

These stereotypes and negative attitudes must be shed by gay men before they can develop a sense of pride and positive self-image. While most prejudicial statements concerning "gayness" may be consciously rejected by those successfully formulating a gay identity, some are less consciously perceived. Unconscious beliefs of personal failure, unhappiness, relational impermanence, or unrecognized beliefs in heteronormative constructions of "natural" may be especially detrimental to gay male identity and coupling.

Problems regarding internalized homophobia are described by Forstein (1986, p. 114), who writes, "Although many gay people aspire to 'couplehood,' their capacity to function and grow within the context of an intimate relationship is significantly determined by the degree to which a positive self-affirming gay identity has been formed." Isay (1989, p. 92) argues that gay men establishing intimate relationships have, at least in part, integrated a healthy gay identity. He writes, "The capacity [for gay men] to fall in love and to maintain a healthy relationship over time requires a high degree of self-esteem, or 'healthy narcissism'. . . . Only a man with a healthy sense of self-esteem can feel capable of being loved and of loving." It may be hypothesized that a minimal level of self-acceptance must exist before a gay man might even entertain the notion of same-sex relational involvement, but this does not imply that internalized homophobia is absent in even the healthiest of gay male relationships as a consequence of growing up within the dominant heterosexist culture.

Heterosexism may be defined as the blatant cultural disavowal of the validity of same-sex desire and coupling. While internalized homophobia describes the absorption of negative social attitudes, heterosexism creates the social structure of gay invisibility. Describing this phenomenon, Blumenfeld and Raymond (1988, p. 244) state,

> When parents automatically expect that their children will marry a person of the other sex at some future date and will rear children within this union; when the only possible and satisfying relationships portrayed by the media are heterosexual; when teachers presume all of their students are straight and teach only about the contributions of heterosexuals—these are examples of heterosexism. It takes the form of pity—when the dominant group looks upon sexual minorities as poor unfortunates who "can't help being the way they are."

Heterosexism is institutionalized in the United States through the lack of national legal protection for gay men and lesbians. Same-sex behavior in over half of the states remains illegal, and gay men and lesbians are predominantly excluded from protection regulating housing discrimination, fair employment practices, immigration, child custody rights, adoption, inheritance, security clearance, approved participation in the military, and police protection. Gay male relationships are not open to legal recognition, denying same-sex couples the economic advantages of marriage. Perhaps most profound, however, is the lack of rituals, models, sanctioned boundaries, and cultural support for gay coupling, making explicit society's view that gay male relationships are not "real," or equal to those of heterosexuals (Meyer, 1990).

The lack of societal support for gay male relationships is often painfully brought home through the intolerance or disrespect of family members toward a gay son's partner. Some parents and siblings may respond favorably to one's relationship. However, for almost all, coming out to parents and relatives in regard to one's same-sex relationship is a time of significant stress. McWhirter and Mattison (1984, p. 240), in their study of gay male couples, found that the majority of their subjects did not have full family support or participation. They reported,

> Many have a warm relationship with one set of parents and no relationship with the other. In other cases the families are unaware of or disregard their son's sexual orientation. These

men return to their respective homes at holiday times and on other occasions of family celebrations without their partners.

A lack of familial support for gay relationships may weigh heavily upon the couple. Expectations of continuing family of origin involvement and the maintenance of prior family roles may persist, promoting relational conflict and stress. Family rejection may reinforce internalized homophobia and may also color perceptions of self and relational value. For others, family rejection may promote a profound sense of isolation.

COUPLING DYNAMICS

McWhirter and Mattison's (1984; 1985; 1988) monumental work on gay male couples presents a stage model that is longitudinal and is conceptualized as an aid in describing and understanding male couples formation. McWhirter and Mattison's work emphasizes stages of gay male coupling. "Stage One" dynamics are characterized by high limerance (compatibility) and cohesion. As the relationship becomes more reality-based and conflicts surface, the couple may begin to withdraw from each other. They suggest that fear of intimacy in "Stage One" couples may also promote emotional withdrawal. Should couples survive this process, "Stage Two" issues and themes occur. "Stage Two" is described as a period when passion declines and conflict is based on differences in values and tastes. McWhirter and Mattison also suggest that "Stage Two" couples must begin to address the issue of exclusivity/nonexclusivity, and jealousy or possessiveness is common. Problems in "Stage Three" center around increased needs for autonomy and the concomitant experience of loss of early romanticism, with independent functioning by one member of the couple often perceived as a threat generating anxiety or anger. "Stage Four" is depicted as "a time of considerable distancing from each other." In "Stage Five," after ten to twenty years together, "routine and monotony" become causes of distress for gay male couples. McWhirter and Mattison (1988, p. 250) write that the "tendency to become more fixed or rigid in personality characteristics while struggling to change each other can also plague men who have been together over ten years."

Couples in "Stage Six" reportedly express feelings of "restless-ness, sometimes withdrawal and feelings of aimlessness," often as a function of the attainment of both individual and coupling goals.

McWhirter and Mattison's stage theory of gay male coupling seems to overemphasize structural disengagement and open cou-pling dynamics for all but those engaged in early coupling forma-tion. However, that gay male couples must be understood as vary-ing according to life transitions and an understanding of relational stages are both crucial to normalizing conflicts in gay couples, allowing for an appreciation of differences, conflicts, or dissatisfac-tions to be more a function of stage sequence, rather than inherent to the relationship.

While an assessment of stage development is essential to ap-propriate descriptions of gay male couples, it too must be tied to the effects of internalized homophobia. Couple formation requires the creation and maintenance of boundaries (Johnson and Keren, 1996). The level of permeability of boundaries may be influenced by that which is perceived as threatening to the couple. Couples may react to anticipated or actual responses of familial rejection, peer indifference to the meaning of partnership, and/or internalized negativity by producing closed coupling systems as an attempt to exclude social hostility and fortify the "bonds of love." Thus, this style of coupling may be understood as an adaptive reaction to cultural conditions. The greater the level of perceived threat, the more closed a relationship may become. Yet closed coupling sys-tems generate tremendous pressure on the couple, making partners feel responsible for fulfilling a predominance of the other partner's needs. Without cultural sanctions against coupling dissolution, or social support to reduce relational pressures, gay male couples may move from markedly enmeshed, to disengaged, to dissolved, to newly formed and enmeshed relationships.

Alternatively, internalized homophobia may promote highly dis-engaged coupling styles as a consequence of absorbed devaluing of same-sex intimacy. Gay male couples who adopt a "best friend" or "roommate" model of coupling may establish extremely loose rela-tional boundaries (open relational style) as a manifestation of social/ familial hostility, or internalized and unconscious attitudes concern-ing the "impossibility" of gay male relations. In extreme forms, the disconnectedness of highly open boundaries (closed relational style) makes relational involvement irrelevant, again potentiating coupling dissolution.

While neither open nor closed relational styles, in themselves, are indicative of future relational failure, the level of adaptability of these systems to respond to conflict becomes crucial. Both chaotic and rigid coupling styles may lack the skills to alter relational patterns in order to address conflicts arising from or occurring within extreme forms of open or closed systems. Again, coupling adaptability may be influenced by internalized homophobia. For those who once sought and anchored themselves to societal rules as a means of avoiding exposure, suppressing desire, or "fitting in," rigidity may become a way of life. Forstein (1986, p. 113) states, "The more conflicted a gay man is about his homosexuality, the more rigid and stereotyped his gender role identity is likely to be." For others, maintaining chaotic decision-making styles may allow for an avoidance of commitment, initiated by an earlier avoidance to commit to a gay identity and lifestyle. Although structural paradigms are always affected by parental modeling, this does not preclude the importance of homophobia in influencing structural dynamics in gay male couples.

Other theorists have focused on issues of sexuality and sexual dysfunction in gay male couples. Shernoff, in his notable work with gay male couples, presents a classification system in which he examines a variety of relationship styles (Shernoff, 1995). He develops five categories with which to define male couples: (1) the sexually exclusive couple; (2) the sexually nonexclusive but unacknowledged open relationship; (3) the primarily sexually exclusive relationship; (4) the sexually nonexclusive and acknowledged open relationship; and (5) nonsexual lovers.

While Shernoff's model has grown out of his extensive work with gay men and gay male couples, this model may have limitations to a social work practitioner who has had fewer opportunities to work with gay male couples. Practitioners may find themselves, in using this model, which constructs gay male coupling around sexuality and sexual behaviors, unwittingly presuming that sex is the exclusive area around which gay men partner. To an unseasoned or nongay practitioner, this model may reproduce the stereotype about gay male identity and gay males coupling as defined primarily by their sexuality.

In another important contribution to the literature on gay male couples, George and Behrendt (1988) suggest that sexual dysfunction in one or both partners may produce stress on the couple, and they state that, anecdotally, many gay male couples are never asked about this. They hypothesize that this is due to a provider's lack of comfort with the subject or their misperception that gay male couples do not experience sexual dysfunction. They break out the concept of sexual dysfunction into three areas: (1) inhibited sexual desire; (2) inhibited male orgasm; and (3) inhibited sexual excitement. Inhibited sexual desire, they suggest, may be caused by either internalized cultural homophobia or a phobic aversion to sex generally. Inhibited orgasm may also be due to internal conflicts related to homophobia or sexual fantasies of aggression and the fear of loss of control. Lastly, inhibited sexual excitement is considered a result of discrepant views of masculinity perpetuated by society, which results in the belief that their performance is being "graded" by their partner, leading to inhibition.

MALE GENDER ROLE SOCIALIZATION

It has been argued (Finnegan and McNally, 1987; Johnson and Keren, 1996; Mass, 1990) that gay men, like heterosexual men, are socialized to behave within culturally determined gender patterns. While some gay men may believe themselves to have rejected conditioning associated with socially determined masculine role norms, often heterosexually prescribed masculine values are latent. These values may include themes of power and control. While any relationship, regardless of gender and sexual orientation, must address these issues, male socialization, in its emphasis on winning and competition, makes male intimacy especially problematic.

In addition to problems associated with masculine identity, any subgroup that has been culturally marginalized or disempowered will have a greater likelihood to act out their social repression through intimate relationships. This may be particularly salient in gay men, where attempts at self-control over one's same-sex desires in early stages of gay identity formation and fears of exposure are apparent. Cabaj (1991, p. 2), in regard to help seeking in gay men, states, "Since men, in general, and gay men who are struggling to accept their homosexuality, in particular, have difficulties with intimacy and sharing, they may seek help to learn how to communicate about and be comfortable with intimacy." Thus, the manifestation of power dynamics interrupting the potential for intimate relations in gay male couples may be more a function of internalized homophobia rather than, or exclusively, masculine gender socialization. This social hypothesis would also predict that the observation of issues of power and control in gay male couples may be more extreme in those less integrated in their gay male identities and community.

JOINING

Before couples counseling can become solution focused, the social worker must join with the couple in a therapeutic alliance. This requires that the social work practitioner is perceived as both nonjudgmental and supportive of the couple. For many gay male couples, suspiciousness of helping professionals and the profession of social work in general due to homophobia may predict the delay or avoidance of initiating treatment. There is a history in the mental health profession of viewing homosexuality as psychopathological with curative therapies existing to treat the condition (Isay, 1989). According to George and Behrendt (1988, p. 78), "Homosexual men will seek therapy when they recognize they are having difficulties as a couple, provided that (a) identifying themselves as a couple is not precluded by discriminatory practices by the therapist, and (b) they are not treated as if their homosexuality were the cause of their conflict." Similar to other minority populations, gay male couples integrated into the gay male community may be more likely to turn to friends in times of crisis as opposed to social work practitioners because of fears of provider prejudice (Hines and Boyd-Franklin, 1982), as well as gender socialization concerning male attitudes of self-sufficiency and the rationalization of feelings (Isensee, 1990).

Should services be sought, however, gay male couples are often particularly sensitive to bias on the part of the social work provider. Many gay male couples will only contact gay or lesbian therapists to avoid potential insensitivity. For gay male clients engaging in treatment with someone unknown to the lesbian/gay community, direct questioning of the social worker about homosexuality and personal sexual orientation is common. Such questioning, however, could lead to initial engagement problems as an inquiry process by the therapist may cause stress for the clients who may feel resentful that they have had to "educate" the therapist about gay couples. Additionally, some gay male couples may feel reluctant to question the therapist, and instead, maintain an initial suspension of trust. Without direct attention to issues of trust, sexual orientation, and a respect for differences between heterosexual providers and gay male clients, treatment progress and at the very least initial the initial engagement process may be significantly impaired.

The issue of trust for gay male couples working with heterosexual providers is magnified for couples experiencing problems of internalized homophobia. Couples struggling with culturally absorbed negativity may project these attitudes onto the social work practitioner. However, it should be understood that initial defensive posturing may be expressed by any gay male couple engaging in services with heterosexual or gay providers, and would not, in itself, reveal unusual coupling dynamics.

Self-disclosure by gay male social work practitioners is essential in counseling gay male couples due to role modeling and self-empowerment (Kooden, 1991). Gay male couples who seek services from a gay male practitioner who refuses to acknowledge his sexual orientation for reasons of professional "neutrality" may perceive the practitioner's decision as problematic and often as a homophobic practice in reproducing the psychosocial stressors of the closet.

ASSESSING PRESENTING CONCERNS

The assessment of presenting concerns by clients and social workers is filtered by both theory and unconscious assumptions. Social work practitioners working with gay male couples must continuously assess countertransferential dynamics influencing perceptions of the couple, as well as interpretations and interventions. One must be particularly careful about attributing coupling dynamics to internal dysfunctioning, rather than attending to social and systemic conditions influencing relational patterns. Normalizing and reframing coupling conflict through attributions of stage level, heterosexism, internalized homophobia, structural paradigm, and gender socialization often provide gay male couples with an opportunity to escape self and partner blaming for problems. This will in turn provide clients and the practitioner with a working alliance by communicating that the provider understands the unique conditions affecting the gay male couple and is not interested in pathologizing them.

INTERVENTIONS

Systems theory and intervention act to reestablish relational homeostasis through conflict resolution without presenting dysfunctional symptoms. This requires an analysis of communication patterns, triangles, hierarchies, roles, and boundaries (Carl, 1990). While systems theory makes irrelevant the sexual orientation of the couple, some systems providers may be biased in their approach to gay male couples. For example, therapists working with couples with one or both partners who are living with HIV/AIDS may discourage multiple sexual contacts, regardless of the couple's valuing of nonexclusive sexual involvements. This may stem from a belief that nonexclusivity interferes with coupling intimacy, or as a reaction to fears of HIV transmission (Goldenberg and Goldenberg, 1990; Odets and Shernoff, 1995). A second example of provider bias is the devaluing of relational role definition by social workers imposing personal values of role fluidity. These examples of provider bias reflect a superimposition of heteronormativity onto individual gay couples, rather than respecting a diversity of coupling styles. Given the dearth of information and training on systemic interventions with gay male couples, provider bias is somewhat understandable. However, it behooves social work practitioners to appreciate the values and uniqueness of any couple with whom one works.

CASE ILLUSTRATION

Tom and David were self-referred for couples work with presenting concerns of emotional disengagement on Tom's part, described by David, and Tom stating that he wasn't sure he was capable of "loving anyone." Through the assessment process, it was learned that Tom and David had been together for three years. According to McWhirter and Mattison's (1984) stage model, they were reacting within the context of the "Nesting Stage," with common difficulties of developing compatibility, and dealing with relational ambivalence after the initial "blending" period. They reported nonsexual relations for six months, and Tom heatedly reported finding David to be using "phone sex" lines with increasing regularity. David felt sympathetic to Tom, but was unsure if he could assure Tom that he could discontinue this behavior. David also reported that their initial sexual life together had been the best he had ever known, but over the last year he felt he had just "lost interest." This loss of coupling eroticism and sexuality appeared to be related to a period of significant stress and depression for David during a job change. It was at that time that David had become increasingly withdrawn.

David reported that his relationship with Tom was his first gay relationship, while Tom had had one prior partner of six years. Tom reported that the relationship had ended for many of the same reasons he felt he and David were experiencing difficulties: lack of emotional and sexual contact, problems communicating, and the feeling that David "just didn't care." The latter issue was further reinforced by David's recent trip home for the holidays, leaving Tom behind because he was not "out" to his parents. Tom expressed some understanding of David's reluctance to come out to his parents who are devoutly religious, but with further exploration bitterly complained about David's disregard for his needs.

As the couple was informed of the normality of their conflicts as a function of coupling development, they visibly relaxed. However, when it was also suggested that both David and Tom were contributing to their relational problems, rather than David alone, Tom became increasingly anxious. Yet this also facilitated the exploration of Tom's occasionally demanding attitude and lack of empathy regarding David's emotional concerns that left David to fend for himself and led both partners to become increasingly angry and polarized.

Over time, it was discovered that David's sexual difficulty with Tom was largely a function of internalized homophobia. They both began to explore their histories of shame surrounding their desires and came to realize how both partners shared in the problem of closeness. These discussions produced a depth of intimacy between them previously unrealized and soon they began, tentatively, to return to their prior sexual involvement. While Tom and David continue to address communication problems and a tendency to disengage when stressed, they have been able to solidify their partnership through support. Their acceptance of the social worker's interventions was founded upon the worker's respect for the couples' strengths, validation of their homoerotic and intimacy needs, and theoretical appreciation of both gay-specific and general systems dynamics impacting upon coupling development.

IMPLICATIONS FOR SOCIAL WORK PRACTICE

Ecologically oriented social workers who are interested in working with gay couples should be prepared to consider the following:

- As one undertakes an assessment process, the basis for the referral or the presenting problem must be prioritized and respected, rather than any predetermined agenda on the part of the social work provider (Compton and Galloway, 1989; Hepworth and Larsen, 1990; Meyer, 1993). It is important to remember that gay male couples may be somewhat reserved during an initial contact until it has been established that the provider is accepting of the couple's sexual orientation and nonjudgmental with regard to their concerns.
- Environmental stressors often precipitate relational distress and can lead to maladaptive coping by one or by both members of the couple. Responses to environmental stressors need to be appreciated within the context of the unique strengths, histories, and needs of each member of any gay male partnership.
- In addition to assessing the unique characteristics of the couple, social work practitioners should be trained in both general systems theory, gay male coupling, and gay male developmental dynamics, as well as becoming knowledgeable about social and cultural factors impacting upon gay men. Unless comfortable with this knowledge base, it is recommended that the provider make an appropriate referral.
- Practitioners need to address levels of internalized homophobia within each partner. Due to internalized homophobia, het-

erosexism, and negative media depictions of gay men, gay males in a couple may believe that relationships are difficult or impossible to sustain and may believe that they should define their relationships around their sexual behavior, gender constructions, or cultural stereotypes rather than discovering the meaning of their own partnership. It is often very helpful to assist gay couples in analyzing these belief systems and how they may negatively affect their relationships.

• Practitioners should assess at what stage each partner and the relational system is in the coming out process. George and Behrendt (1988) identify the coming out process as unfolding in three ways: (1) acknowledgement of one's own self as gay (private admission); (2) acknowledging one's identity to other people and building a support system; and (3) acknowledging one's sexual orientation to co-workers, relatives, and hetero-sexual friends, which can be considered a high risk for rejection. All of these may produce significant stress for the couple.

• Practitioners need to assess the extent of social supports. Many gay male couples stop socializing within gay male communities, finding support from each other. During crises, they may experience social isolation. Gay male couples in crisis may need to expand social networks.

• Depending on prior negative experiences with people in positions of authority, including social service providers, homophobia may be anticipated and projected onto the provider. Unless these transferential issues are addressed, progress in treatment may be greatly compromised.

• HIV/AIDS and other sexually transmitted diseases have significantly affected gay men. Social work practitioners need to reassure clients about confidentiality and inquire about HIV fears, exposures, infection, or diagnosis of AIDS. Just as individual gay men will require interventions that are differentiated across the HIV continuum (HIV ignorance and ongoing high-risk behavior, HIV untested, HIV negative, HIV positive and asymptomatic, HIV symptomatic, diagnosed with AIDS, terminally ill and dying as a result of AIDS) so too will gay male couples require differentiated interventions depending upon each part-

ner's HIV status. (Cadwell, Burnham, and Forstein, 1994; Carl, 1990; Livingston, 1995, 1996; Odets and Shernoff, 1995).
• Given the reported higher rates of chemical dependency among gay men, assessment of substance use, abuse, and dependency, and referrals to gay-affirmative treatment programs is essential (Finnegan and McNally, 1987; Faltz, 1988, 1992; Greene and Faltz, 1991; Ratner, 1988; Weinberg, 1994).

CONCLUSION

Social work practice with gay male couples within an ecosystemic perspective has similarities to work with nongay couples as well as distinctions from heterocentric interventions and heterosexist treatment. Effective interventions with gay male couples requires an appreciation of the interactions among cultural oppression, coupling dynamics, and individual development. Most important, social work practice with gay male couples mandates a respect for intimate unions in any form.

REFERENCES

Biery, R. E. (1990). *Understanding homosexuality. The pride and the prejudice.* Austin: Edward-William Publishing Company.

Blumenfeld, W. J. and Raymond, D. (1988). *Looking at gay and lesbian life.* Boston: Beacon Press.

Bozett, F. W. and Sussman, M. B. (Eds.). (1990). *Homosexuality and family relations.* Binghamton, NY: Harrington Park Press.

Cabaj, R. P. (1991 April). Counseling gay couples. *Focus. A Guide to AIDS Research and Counseling, 6*(5): San Francisco, CA: UCSF AIDS Health Project.

Cadwell, S. A., Burnham, R. A., and Forstein, M. (Eds.). (1994). *Therapists on the front line. Psychotherapy with gay men in the age of AIDS.* Washington, DC: American Psychiatric Press.

Carl, D. (1990). *Counseling same-sex couples.* New York and London: W.W. Norton and Company.

Compton, B. R. and Galloway, B. (1989). *Social work processes,* fourth edition. Belmont, CA: Wadsworth Publishing Company.

Faltz, B. G. (1988). Substance abuse and the lesbian and gay community: Assessment and intervention. In M. Shernoff and W. Scott (Eds.), *The sourcebook on lesbian and gay health care,* second edition (pp. 151-161). Washington, DC: National Lesbian and Gay Health Foundation.

Faltz, B. G. (1992). Counseling chemically dependent lesbians and gay men. In S. H. Dworkin and F. J. Gutierrez (Eds.), *Counseling gay men and lesbians: Journey to the end of the rainbow* (pp. 245-258). Alexandria, VA: American Counseling Association.

Finnegan, D. G. and McNally, E. B. (1987). *Dual identities. Counseling chemically dependent gay men and lesbians.* Center City, MN: Hazelden.

Forstein, M. (1986). Psychodynamic psychotherapy with gay male couples. In T. S. Stein and C. J. Cohen (Eds.), *Contemporary perspectives on psychotherapy with lesbians and gay men* (pp. 103-137). New York and London: Plenum Medical Book Company.

George, K. D. and Behrendt, A. E. (1988). Therapy for male couples experiencing relationship problems and sexual problems. In E. Coleman (Ed.), *Integrated identity for gay men and lesbians. Psychotherapeutic approaches for emotional well-being* (pp. 77-88). Binghamton, NY: Harrington Park Press.

Goldenberg, H. and Goldenberg, I. (1990). *Counseling today's families.* Pacific Grove, CA: Brooks/Cole Publishing Company.

Greene, D. and Faltz, B. (1991). Chemical dependency and relapse in gay men with HIV infection: Issues and treatment. In M. Shernoff (Ed.), *Counseling chemically dependent people with HIV illness* (pp. 79-90). Binghamton, NY: The Haworth Press.

Hartman, A. (1996). Social policy as a context for lesbian and gay families: The political is personal. In J. Laird and R-J. Green (Eds.), *Lesbians and gays in couples and families. A handbook for therapists* (pp. 69-85). San Francisco: Jossey-Bass.

Hepworth, D. H. and Larsen, J. A. (1990). *Direct social work practice,* third edition. Belmont, CA: Wadsworth Publishing Company.

Hines, P. M. and Boyd-Franklin, N. (1982). Black families. In M. McGoldrick, J. K. Pearce, and J. Giordano (Eds.), *Ethnicity and family therapy* (pp. 84-107). New York and London: Guilford Press.

Isay, R. A. (1989). *Being homosexual: Gay men and their development.* New York: Avon Books.

Isensee, R. (1990). *Love between men: Enhancing intimacy and keeping your relationship alive.* New York: Simon and Schuster.

Isensee, R. (1991). *Growing up gay in a dysfunctional family: A guide for gay men reclaiming their lives.* New York: Prentice Hall.

Johnson, T. W. and Keren, M. S. (1996). Creating and maintaining boundaries in male couples. In J. Laird and R-J. Green (Eds.), *Lesbians and gays in couples and families. A handbook for therapists* (pp. 231-250). San Francisco, CA: Jossey-Bass.

Kooden, H. (1991). Self-disclosure: The gay male therapist as agent of social change. In C. Silverstein (Ed.), *Gays, lesbians, and their therapists* (pp. 143-154). New York: W. W. Norton.

Livingston, D. (1995). Group counseling for gay couples coping with AIDS. In W. Odets and M. Shernoff (Eds.), *The second decade of AIDS: A mental health practice handbook* (pp. 69-84). New York: Hatherleigh Press.

Livingston, D. (1996). A systems approach to AIDS counseling for gay couples. In M. Shernoff (Ed.), *Human services for gay people: Clinical and community practice* (pp. 83-93). Binghamton, NY: The Haworth Press.

Malyon, A. K. (1985). Psychotherapeutic implications of internalized homophobia in gay men. In J. C. Gonsiorek (Ed.), *A guide to psychotherapy with gay and lesbian clients* (pp. 59-69). Binghamton, NY: Harrington Park Press.

Mass, L. D. (1990). *Homosexuality and sexuality: Dialogues of the sexual revolution, volume I.* Binghamton, NY: Harrington Park Press.

McGoldrick, M. (1996). Foreword. In J. Laird and R-J. Green (Eds.), *Lesbians and gays in couples and families: A handbook for therapists* (pp. xi-xiv). San Francisco, CA: Jossey-Bass.

McWhirter, D. P. and Mattison, A. M. (1984). *The male couple: How relationships develop.* Englewood Cliffs, NJ: Prentice-Hall.

McWhirter, D. P. and Mattison, A. M. (1985). Psychotherapy for gay male couples. In J. C. Gonsiorek (Ed.), *A guide to psychotherapy with gay and lesbian clients* (pp. 79-91). Binghamton, NY: Harrington Park Press.

McWhirter, D. P. and Mattison, A. M. (1988). Stage discrepancy in male couples. In E. Coleman (Ed.), *Integrated identity for gay men and lesbians: Psychotherapeutic approaches for emotional well-being* (pp. 89-99). Binghamton, NY: Harrington Park Press.

Meyer, C. H. (1993). *Assessment in social work practice.* NY: Columbia University Press.

Meyer, J. (1990). Guess who's coming to dinner this time? A study of gay intimate relationships and the support for those relationships. In F. W. Bozett and M. B. Sussman (Eds.), *Homosexuality and family relations* (pp. 59-82). Binghamton, NY: Harrington Park Press.

Moses, A. E. and Hawkins, R. O., Jr. (1986). *Counseling lesbian women and gay men: A life-issues approach.* Columbus, OH: Merrill Publishing Company.

Odets, W. and Shernoff, M. (Eds.) (1995). *The second decade of AIDS: A mental health practice handbook.* New York: Hatherleigh Press.

Ratner, E. (1988). Treatment issues for chemically dependent lesbians and gay men. In M. Shernoff and W. Scott (Eds.), *The sourcebook on lesbian and gay health care,* second edition (pp. 162-168). Washington, DC: National Lesbian and Gay Health Foundation.

Rothberg, B. and Weinstein, D. L. (1996). A primer on lesbian and gay families. In M. Shernoff (Ed.), *Human services for gay people: Clinical and community practice* (pp. 55-68). Binghamton, NY: The Haworth Press.

Savin-Williams, R. C. (1990). *Gay and lesbian youth: Expressions of identity.* Washington, DC: Hemisphere.

Shernoff, M. (1995). Male couples and their relationship styles. *Journal of Gay & Lesbian Social Services, 2*(2), 43-57.

Weinberg, G. (1972). *Society and the healthy homosexual.* Garden City, NY: Anchor Press/Doubleday.

Weinberg, T. S. (1994). *Gay men, drinking, and alcoholism.* Carbondale and Edwardsville, IL: Southern Illinois University Press.

Chapter 10

Social Work Practice with Gay Men and Lesbians Within Communities

Joyce Hunter
Gerald P. Mallon

Although the singular concept of "the gay and lesbian community" is a myth, because in actuality there are numerous lesbian and gay communities, each reflecting the diversity that exists in the population (Boykin, 1996; Chan, 1989; Espin, 1987; Loiacano, 1989), the notion of practicing with lesbians and gay men within communities is an essential ingredient for anyone interested in developing a foundation of knowledge about this group. With its web of internal relationships among individuals, families, and other collectivities, and its complex of relationships to the world outside itself, communities should always be one of the focal points of the social worker's attention when working with lesbian and gay persons.

One conceptual framework used throughout this text that is helpful for further development of understanding array of practice issues in working with lesbians and gay men is an ecological perspective. The ecological metaphor, posed by Germain (1985) and others (Germain and Gitterman, 1996; Meyer, 1976), suggested that the community is an integral part of the life space of individuals and collectivities that we serve. The transactional nature of ecological concepts central to this framework do not refer to persons or environments alone, but symbolize a relationship between them. The concepts of adaptedness, stress, coping, competence, self-direction, relatedness to others and to the natural world, and self-esteem are all applicable within a community context.

PRACTICE WITH COMMUNITIES
WITHIN AN ECOLOGICAL FRAMEWORK

Adaptedness and adaptation are appropriate concepts to use in considering the lesbian and gay community or any other human collectivity. For the social worker who is ecologically oriented, the community's exchanges with its external environment and its internal environment are also a part of the unit of attention. Although it is not appropriate to say that a community experiences stress, individuals within the community do. Lesbians and gay men, because they have had to live their lives within the context of a hostile environment, have experienced a disproportionate amount of shared stress. Consequently, it is appropriate to say that as a community, lesbian and gay persons have experienced high levels of community stress. The overwhelming presence of such stressful conditions may be considered as the outcome of a community's transactions with the larger environment that produces social pollutants, oppression, and discrimination.

Living within a societal environment that promotes stress and is hostile to their very existence causes many lesbian and gay persons to search for ways to cope with what Goffman (1963) would call their "spoiled" identity. "Physical and social environments," notes Germain (1978, p. 540), "may fail to provide the protection, security, and the biological, cognitive, social and emotional nutriments individuals, families, and groups need." When communities fail to provide such nourishment, which one would need to sustain life, its members, in this case lesbians and gay men, must almost continually make adjustments and adaptations.

DISEMPOWERMENT AND SOCIAL POLLUTION

Although lesbians and gay persons essentially face all the conventional stressors of life, they also encounter some that are unique to their status as marginalized individuals in society. As such, adaptations are necessary to achieve a "goodness of fit" between the person:environment. It is this dilemma that serves as the theoretical framework for understanding lesbian and gay persons in a community context.

Indeed, it is the Western culture's belief system that supports the negative myths, stereotypes, and misconceptions about lesbian and gay persons, and not the orientation itself that is a major life stressor for lesbians and gay persons. People who are perceived as "other" are frequently denied power and privileges granted to others in the majority. Withholding of power by dominant groups from other groups on the basis of personal or cultural features, called coercive power; as well as the abuse of power by dominant groups that creates technological pollution, endangering the health and well-being of people and communities, known as exploitative power, are two contemporary ecological concepts presented by Germain and Gitterman (1996) in their revised text of the life model. These concepts have particular relevance to the experiences of lesbians and gay persons because disempowerment and social pollution are expressions of the destructive relationships between persons and environments and, as such, impose enormous adaptive tasks on oppressed populations.

When a poor fit is present, as evidenced by the presence of disempowering mechanisms and social pollutants, persons may choose one of three adaptations: (1) they may attempt to change themselves; (2) they may attempt to change their environment; or (3) they may attempt to change the person:environment relationship in order to achieve an improved fit (Germain and Gitterman, 1996). In earlier work, Germain (1981) and Hartmann (1958) presented a variation on this third adaptive strategy, calling it "migration." Such a designation, which is a strategy that clearly resonates with the experiences of many lesbian and gay individuals who have relocated from rural and suburban environs to urban "gay/lesbian affirming" communities, suggests that a good fit could be obtained by relocating to a more nurturing environment. Such individuals leave their families, leave their homes, and migrate to large urban areas that provide the illusion of safety at worst, and the promise of community at best.

THE SEARCH FOR COMMUNITY WITHIN THE CONTEXT OF THE COMING-OUT PROCESS

The development of the lesbian and gay community may also be viewed within the context of the coming-out process. Coming out, which has been conceptualized by researchers and practitioners

(Cass, 1979; Coleman, 1981; Minton and McDonald, 1984; Troiden, 1993) as a developmental framework that unfolds in stages, may also be a useful model in viewing lesbians and gay men within the context of community. One four-stage model, incorporating and elaborating on other previous models, is proposed by Troiden (1993). Troiden identifies the first stage as *sensitization,* which is characterized by a general feeling of being marginal and different from others. This stage is followed by *identity confusion,* in which individuals think that they might be lesbian or gay, but are unable to decide. In the third stage, *identity assumption,* individuals can begin to identify themselves as lesbian or gay. The final stage, *commitment,* culminates in the development of positive feelings about being lesbian or gay as individuals begin to incorporate this identity into other social and personal arenas. As the following case example illustrates, initial engagement with the lesbian and gay community is a natural part of the coming-out process.

> John is a twenty-eight-year old Caucasian gay male who recently came to live in New York City. He came to New York from St. Louis, Missouri, to accept a new employment situation. John was not out in St. Louis, but viewed coming to New York as an opportunity to live his life as a gay man more openly. After establishing himself in his new job and finding an affordable habitat, John sought out the "gay community" in New York. Initially, like most gay men and lesbians who come to New York, John spent a great deal of his free time in Greenwich Village. Since John did not drink or smoke, he spent little time in the well-known gay bars in the community; instead he sought to find other men like him in some of the various groups that met at the Lesbian and Gay Community Services Center. Although John was initially unnerved by the wide variety of groups they offered, within a few weeks, he found his niche. He signed up with a gay softball league, volunteered at a gay and lesbian youth service agency, and began the empowering process of developing a sense of community with others who were like him.

As a lesbian or gay person deals with issues concerning whether or not to be open about lesbian or gay sexual orientation, one must make adaptations. Adaptive exchanges that support and release human potential, growth, health, and satisfaction are viewed as positive and affirming of one's identity. Dysfunctional exchanges that fail to support adaptiveness and may interfere with the potential for adaptiveness are viewed as maladaptive. Ultimately, maladaptive exchanges can lead to an unfavorable fit. However, it is important to note that the degree of adaptiveness between a person and his or her environment is not fixed: the relationship between them is constantly changing in large and small ways.

It is probably similarly inaccurate to say that a community copes or fails to cope with stress, as it is the individual members of the community who experience stress. When a community experiences stress, we are likely to see a community that is demoralized, alienated, helpless, or disorganized. In some instances, needed resources that are available to other communities may have been withheld by the larger environment. In other instances, a member's coping efforts may be viewed as problematic behaviors because the observer's professional or personal value orientations act either to obscure the cultural base of the member's coping style or to block recognition of the coping strengths in the context of a hostile environment. Germain (1985) notes that two ecological concepts, already alluded to in the vignette presented above, shed further light on these issues: the concepts of habitat and niche.

HABITAT

Habitat refers to the place where an individual resides or is found. In the case of lesbians or gay men, it can be a rural, suburban, or urban setting in a way that fits with their life. Functional habitats support the health and social functioning of individuals and are likely to produce or to contribute to feelings of acceptance, belonging, and joy. Dysfunctional habitats are apt to promote feelings of isolation, alienation, and distress. Experiencing stress in habitats may interfere with the basic functions of family and community life. Similarly, experiencing comfort and a place to call home may sustain the individual by providing him or her with the nurturance and nutrition necessary for connection with community. Habitat, then, is a critical arena for all practice with individuals, families, groups, and community or one of its segments. Practitioners must have the knowledge and skill to work in new ways to improve habitats. What follows is an array of situations where habitats may need to be considered as a unit of attention.

A social worker may work with a lesbian or gay individual who is experiencing significant stress in his or her environment by assisting them with locating housing in a gay/lesbian-affirming neighborhood or by helping a new lesbian or gay "migrant" to determine which neighborhoods are affirming toward lesbians and gay men and which are not. In urban areas where housing may not be always affordable, the ecologically oriented social worker should be familiar with lesbian and gay roommate services that can assist new migrants with identifying affordable and safe housing and should be able to direct the client toward newspapers that are known to advertise in lesbian and gay communities. However, spacial-temporal dimensions of habitats must also be considered because intrusions into one's psychological, physical, or social space can generate stress by interfering with community customs, status hierarchies, or natural support systems. In the case of rural lesbians and gay men, social or emotional isolation or physical isolation may be brought on by or intensified by geographic isolation or distance. Within urban environments, particularly for lesbians and gay men who have chosen to live within the context of an urban gay or lesbian ghetto, the converse may be true, as a lesbian or gay individual may be saturated with gay or lesbian community.

HIV/AIDS has had a significant impact on the gay and lesbian community (D'Augelli, 1990; Lloyd and Kuzelewicz, 1995; Paul, Hays, and Coates, 1995), but it has had a particular impact on the area of the habitat in that numerous gay men have returned to the habitats of their families of origin to die. Nowhere in the literature is this more vividly or more movingly observed than in the work of physician Abraham Verghese (1994) in a small town in rural Tennessee. Verghese describes a paradigm that he developed to describe this phenomenon of migration:

> I traced the outline of the entire United States . . . I wanted to locate the places where each patient used to live between 1979 and 1985. This was the period in time when most of them had

contracted infection with the AIDS virus. I culled all the stories . . . for example, the young man who had driven down from New York and come to the Miracle Center and died, he had almost certainly contracted his infection in New York City. The brother of Essie, who had come back from a prolonged residence in Florida . . . Otis Jackson who had lived in San Francisco in the Castro area before returning. I could see a distinct pattern emerging on the larger map of the USA. The paradigm was revealed. (pp. 317-324)

Their collective story spoke of an elaborate migration. The first step in this circuitous migration was a disappearance from home and a period of urban living . . . which was followed by the long voyage back home which ended in death.

A social worker in a rural area may need to assist communities in dealing with community members who have left to live in urban centers and come home to live with their families. Although Verghese's work focused on this phenomenon from the perspective of HIV and AIDS, many lesbians and gay men return to their former communities for a wide variety of reasons. As the lesbian and gay individual has frequently been viewed by other members of their families of origin as single and therefore seemingly without the responsibility of spouses or children, many gay men and lesbians are called upon to return to their communities to care for sick parents. Others return to reclaim their positions in the community after having spent some time in an urban area.

The issue of violence directed both inside and outside of the lesbian and gay community (Hanson, 1996; Herek, 1990; Hunter, 1990) is another important issue for social workers to be aware of and to address. Gay men and lesbians are at risk for violence just by being who they are. There is a perception of safety in seeking refuge in communities that are perceived as safe. There is not necessarily safety in numbers. Issues of personal safety are never far from the minds of most lesbians and gay men as they negotiate their lives within the context of their community habitats. These and other conditions related to time, space, and safety within the habitat are experienced and may require intervention at the community level.

NICHE

A niche refers to the position in the community that is occupied by an individual; that is, as Germain (1985, p. 45) referred to it, "their place in the web of life." Niche refers metaphorically to the status occupied by an individual or group within the social structure and is related to issues of power and oppression. That which is defined as health-promoting and growth supporting is defined differently in various societies. Lesbians and gay men occupy niches that generally do not support their needs and goals—as a direct result of their gay or lesbian sexual orientation, which is devalued by a society that presumes and, indeed as Rich (1983) suggests, insists on "compulsory heterosexuality."

Niche, then, is a critical element in the context of all social work practice. When working at the community level, the ecologically oriented social worker must specifically deal with issues of community empowerment (Gutierrez, 1990; Guttierrez, Alvarez, Nemon, and Lewis, 1996; Gutierrez and Ortega, 1991; Lee, 1994; Simon, 1994; Solomon, 1976; Staples, 1990), supporting community strengths (Saleebey, 1991; Weick and Pope, 1988; Weick, Rapp, Sullivan, and Kisthardt, 1989) and reshaping nonsalutory niches. The adaptive responses of competence, self-direction, relatedness, and self-esteem can also be considered as community strengths or capacities that parallel those of individuals.

The competent community is one in which its component parts are able to collaborate effectively in identifying the problems and needs of the community; can achieve a working consensus on goals and priorities; can agree on ways and means to implement the agreed-upon goals; and can collaborate effectively in the required actions (Germain, 1985). Unlike other oppressed groups that may have a recognized "community leader," the gay and lesbian community has no one individual who acts as leader for the collectivity. Nonetheless, the lesbian and gay community is most competent in dealing with its collective life when it draws upon the strengths of many leaders from its diverse population. Most lesbian and gay community members have problem-solving skills such as verbal, writing, and listening skills; have learned to adapt by developing skills in managing conflict, including collaboration, negotiation, and bargaining (See Vaid, 1995); developed skills in public speaking and in leading discussions and consciousness-raising groups; and technical skills in locating, obtaining, and creating their own resources.

The lesbian and gay community is a self-directed community that values and seeks to mobilize the active participation of all members in matters which concern them individually and which are pertinent to the well-being of the community as a collective. The members of the lesbian and gay community are committed to, and engaged in, protecting the community against threats posed by external forces of power. The community also concerns itself with achieving and maintaining internal strengths as the community itself defines them, including mutual aid systems or folk or natural support systems, and deals with the internal threats posed by the loss or absence of mutual concern, hiding, or respect among the community's component parts. The issue of community self-direction is analogous to issues of empowerment, especially as a sense of power and influence can move individuals and communities from a stance of passivity and despair to a stance of action in areas of life that enable persons to move from individual case to the larger societal cause.

The matter of community identity is a jumbled issue, tangled as it is to matters of definition. The concept of a lesbian and gay community is an ambiguous one, ranging across collectivities as the universal community of all gay men and lesbians to neighborhood or gay and lesbian community service center. The matter of community boundaries as the geographic issues of rural, suburban, and urban life present unique dilemmas for lesbians and gay men. Where the boundary is drawn bears on community identity and pride (self-esteem in individual terms). Without a sense of identity, the community will find it difficult to develop commitment to its self-defined needs and goals.

Community competence, self-direction, and identity rest on human-relatedness, on the sense of belonging, and of being "in place." Relatedness is the essence of community. Relatedness to others and to the physical setting evokes the reciprocity of caring and being cared about. Many communities like the lesbian and gay community have transcended the harshness of their conditions by the operations of their natural helping networks (Delgado and Humm-Delgado,

1982; Gitterman and Shulman, 1986), shared pleasure in music, language, dance, social functions, and other affiliations. A community infused with natural support systems is more likely to be a community that is competent, self-directing, and has a firm sense of identity. The development of more than sixty-five lesbian and gay community services centers across the United States has provided a critical boost to the national efforts of the gay and lesbian community (Lesbian and Gay Community Services Center, 1996-1997).

Community is defined by the institutions it builds and by how we take care of those in need (D'Augelli, 1989, 1990; D'Augelli and Garnets, 1995), what we value, how we define our families, how our relationships are sanctioned and validated by government and churches or synagogues. Lesbians and gay men, like other members of oppressed communities have had to create institutions and organizations to serve as a political, social, and a psychological buffer to the hostility of the dominant culture. The most well-known lesbian and gay communities exist in geographically bounded neighborhoods in several large cities and are usually highly visible, even to those who are not gay or lesbian. Gay and lesbian ghettos—Greenwich Village, particularly Christopher Street—and more recently the Chelsea areas in New York City, The Castro in San Francisco, Dupont Circle in Washington, DC, West Hollywood in Los Angeles, sections of the French Quarter in New Orleans, and Key West in Florida—have been created as habitats for gay men and lesbians.

For lesbians and gay persons of color, there is often conflict with their communities of origin over their homosexuality (see Icard, 1985-1986 for one illustration of this conflict). In addition, lesbian and gay persons of color have also had to deal with racism in the lesbian and gay communities. As noted earlier, the notion of the "gay and lesbian community" is misleading because there is a great deal of diversity between lesbians and gay men. People of color, for example, rarely settle in traditionally white enclaves in white neighborhoods (i.e., the Chelsea area in New York City or The Castro in San Francisco). Rather, they find their "niche" within their own racial or ethnic communities, or away from their homes of origin. For a full discussion of this topic, see Walters (Chapter 3) in this collection.

Krieger (1982) identifies a crucial link in the development of the gay and lesbian community with the emergence of the lesbian-feminist movement. Although Betty Friedan, one of the chief architects of the feminist movement, attempted to marginalize women who identified themselves as women loving women from the feminist movement, the movement had an important influence on many lesbian communities. The development of lesbian communities (Lockard, 1985; Ponse, 1980) was also activated by the women's experiences of sexism within gay male organizations. Women's communities appeared to cluster around a network of nonhierarchical institutions such as coffee houses, women's health clinics, battered women's shelters, rape crisis centers, music festivals, and collectives based on lesbian-feminist politics.

The AIDS pandemic was a major impetus for lesbian and gay community building. Intensified political activity, which came too late for thousands who died of AIDS during the silence and inactivity of the Reagan-Bush era, sought to obtain funding for research and programs to address these critical community needs. AIDS organizations developed rapidly in most urban areas, initiated and funded largely by Caucasian gay men, and many of these organizations have succeedingly been managed by lesbians. The lack of national political leadership, inadequate funding, and increased evidence of discrimination based on sexual orientation and HIV status led to greater militancy and the development of action-oriented groups such as ACT-UP (AIDS Coalition to Unleash Power), Queer Nation, and others (Kramer, 1989; Shilts, 1987).

As the gay male community enters its second decade of living with the AIDS pandemic, gay men are searching for new ways to direct their energies and to create community. Eric Rofes (1996, pp. 262-277) offered the following suggestions for gay men interested in "reviving the tribe" in the 1990s:

1. We must De-AIDS gay identity, community, and culture.
2. The gay political movement must prioritize a broad agenda.
3. The community must begin to discuss sex.
4. Support both separate and mixed spaces for HIV-positive and HIV-negative men.
5. Support gay men's involvement with children and youth.

6. Encourage the celebration of life.
7. Encourage gay men to seek spiritual outlets.
8. Gay men must find opportunities for witnessing.
9. Gay men must be able to explore multiple identities.
10. The gay community must encourage the rebirth of gay identities.
11. The community commitment to combating AIDS must continue.
12. Love between men must be treasured and promoted.

Although mainstream historical perspectives have not always documented the contributions of lesbians and gay men (Chauncey, 1994; Duberman, 1991; Duberman, Vicinus, and Chauncey, 1989; Faderman, 1991), the gay and lesbian community has always been involved in organizing itself around a wide variety of issues (Adam, 1987; D'Emilio, 1983; Katz, 1976; Marcus, 1992). Although it is the Stonewall Rebellion (Duberman, 1993) that most activists point to as the beginning of the modern day gay and lesbian liberation movement, the truth is that there were two other liberation organizations that preceded this event—The Mattachine Society, which was established in 1950, and The Daughters of Bilitis, initiated in 1955. Lesbian and gay communities have always had a keen interest in politics (Shilts, 1982), in religion (Boswell, 1980, 1995), in the military (Berube, 1990; Shilts, 1993), in obtaining civil rights (Duberman, 1993; Vaid, 1995), and in organizing efforts against harassment and violence (Comstock, 1991). The gay and lesbian marches, in 1979, 1987, and in 1993 in Washington, DC, played a major role in community development not only in bringing gay men and lesbians together from all over the country, but in stimulating growth and community-consciousness building in their local communities where they live.

The gay and lesbian "bar scene" is still one of the main places to look for a place to fit in. Although most lesbians and gay men first come out within the context of the bar, as it has historically been one of the few safe places for gay and lesbian people to meet and to have access to the more political lesbian and gay community, it is no longer the only place for lesbians and gay men to come together as community. It is even the place that some people go to start a group or to advertise an event.

Although most lesbians and gay men are unrecognizable to heterosexuals, some gay men and lesbians claim membership within one or more of the various subcultures that exist within the gay and lesbian community. Although a full discussion of the various subcultures within gay and lesbian community goes beyond the scope of this chapter, one group, however, merits attention as they are a group that many uninformed heterosexuals erroneously associate with all gay men and lesbians (See Jay and Young, 1979, for a complete pre-AIDS discussion of gay and lesbian sexuality).

In his book *The Celluloid Closet* the late Vito Russo (1981) examines the images of men and women who are a part of the lesbian and gay community and found that throughout history, gay men and lesbians have been portrayed by the media through degrading and malicious stereotypes. Since in many cases these are the only images that the mainstream culture has of the lesbian and gay community, such likenesses are powerfully ingrained into the collective psyche of most of Western society. These pejorative representations have a particularly damaging effect on the way in which the community is viewed.

THE TRANSGENDERED COMMUNITY

One community whose needs and experiences are frequently linked to gay men and lesbians is men and women who are a part of the transgender spectrum. "Transgender" is an umbrella term encompassing the diversity of gender expression including drag queens and kings, bigenders, crossdressers, transgenderists, and transsexuals (R. Blumenson, Director of the Gender Identity Project, a program of the New York Lesbian and Gay Community Services Center, interview, December 21, 1996). These individuals, many of whom cluster together to form their own communities, are people who find their gender identity—the sense of themselves as male or female—in conflict with their anatomical gender. Some transsexuals may live part time in their self-defined gender. Others desire to live fully in their self-identified gender.

Transgender persons have received a great deal of attention in the media recently but less in terms of real understanding. No matter how many talk shows or hit movies (recent examples include *Bird-*

cage and *The Crying Game*) feature transgender persons, most of Western society continues to view the transgender experience as "abnormal." For many transgendered persons, this results in secrecy, shame, depression, and fear. Such feelings can lead to increased isolation and the adoption of maladaptative coping mechanisms to deal with the stress of living in an environment that not only expects compulsory heterosexuality, but conformity to mandatory gender roles as interpreted by Western society.

In recent years, some social work professionals have recognized that the needs of the transgendered community are similar yet different from the needs of gay and lesbian persons with whom they are frequently united under the banner of sexual minority persons. In order to create greater acceptance and adaptedness to their inner feelings, transgendered persons have begun to create their own community support networks and organizations. In the tradition of many lesbian and gay community centers' commitment to fostering empowerment for lesbians and gay men, some centers across the country have begun to sponsor gender identity projects that offer transgendered individuals a place to discover who they are in an atmosphere of self-acceptance with opportunities to build community.

Although the needs of the transgendered community, important as they are, are beyond the scope of this chapter (See Bornstein, 1994; Burke, 1996; Feinberg, 1993, 1996, for further information), practitioners working with persons from the gay and lesbian community should be aware that they will inevitably also interface with members of the transgender community, whose needs, while seemingly similar, are actually quite different. Practitioners interested in learning more about social work practice with members of the transgender community should familiarize themselves with the work of Wicks (1978) and Levine (1978).

IMPLICATIONS FOR SOCIAL WORK PRACTICE

In attempting to work within communities where lesbians and gay men can find a "fit" that both affirm their lives and promotes health, social workers must be willing to move beyond the stereotypes and mythology that surround the lives of gay men and lesbians (Dulaney and Kelly, 1982). Those who work with gay and lesbian persons must be comfortable addressing issues of homosexuality and be open to developing community strategies, using a variety of approaches, many of which have proven to be useful with other oppressed communities (Guttierrez, Alvarez, Nemon, and Lewis, 1996; Hasenfeld and Chesler, 1987; Kemp, 1995; Kennedy and Davis, 1996; Rivera and Erlich, 1995; Rofes, 1996; Weil, 1986, 1996), designed to address the unique needs of each community.

Ecologically oriented social workers who are interested in working with lesbian and gay communities should be prepared to do the following:

1. To engage in conscious, purposeful, and differential use of themselves as professionals, advocates, and change agents in promoting improvement and change in lesbian and gay communities, and equally be prepared to confront those social policies that affect their clients' welfare
2. To posess a commitment to entering this process with the collaboration of partnership with members of the community
3. To recognize the risks that confront highly vulnerable populations while participating in efforts to change communities and social policies that affect lesbians and gay men
4. To posess a willingness to educate the members of the community, increasing their sense of ownership in community projects and demystify the planning process, and by facilitating a move toward active subjects rather than objects of assessment
5. To posess a willingness to approach the community from the position of "respectful" outsider—one who is willing to abandon the role of expert and to allow the participants to become collaborators in the discovery process
6. To posess a professional commitment to pursuing economic and social justice for diverse and at-risk client populations through community practice
7. To be able to assess the need for advocacy and social action in collaboration with clients in the community
8. To expand one's knowledge base regarding the ways in which the interests, traditions, and expectations of diverse clients with

whom they are working coincide and collide with the interests, traditions, and expectations of relevant community leaders

Most gay men and lesbians are living their lives within the context of a hostile environment because the societal norm is that heterosexuality is the dominant sexual orientation. Negotiating life in a hostile environment undoubtedly produces stress and strain. Although a great deal has been written about the impact of stress on the lives of lesbians and gay men, one must ask the question, if this community has been so stressed, then why have so many lesbians and gay men done so well? Perhaps the research conducted with populations who have experienced high levels of stress suggest some answers. Those individuals who have experienced undue stress, particularly those who band together and form family units, emerge from such stress-filled situations as strong and resilient, as contrasted with those who have been previously described in the literature as "at risk." This metaphor of resilience is appropriate for describing most gay men and lesbians who have come together in communities to support one another.

The fact that so many lesbians and gay men survive and become successful functioning adults is a testament to their resilience. Resilience studies (Aldwin, Levenson, and Spiro, 1994; Brooks, 1994; Compas, Hinden, and Gerhardt, 1995), which have provided data on the benefits of adaptability and perseverance in the face of adversity, suggest that the development of strong familylike communities, similar to those families of creation for lesbians and gay men, provide opportunities for the development of a strong sense of identity and pride in the community. Perhaps social workers would do better to foster resilience within gay and lesbian communities rather than to look for the deficiencies that bind groups together.

REFERENCES

Adam, B. (1987). *The making of the gay and lesbian movement.* Boston: Twayne Publishers.

Aldwin, C. M., Levenson, M. R., and Spiro, A. (1994). Vulnerability and resilience to combat exposure: Can stress have lifelong effects. *Psychology and Aging, 9,* 34-44.

Bérubé, A. (1990). *Coming out under fire: The history of lesbian and gay men in World War Two.* New York: The Free Press.

Blumenson, R. (1996 December 21). Personal interview.

Bornstein, K. (1994). *Gender outlaw.* New York: Vintage.

Boswell, J. (1980). *Christianity, social tolerance, and homosexuality.* Chicago: University of Chicago Press.

Boswell, J. (1995). *Same-sex unions in premodern Europe.* New York: Vintage Books.

Boykin, K. (1996). *One more river to cross.* New York: Anchor Books.

Brooks, R. B. (1994). Children at risk: Fostering resilience and hope. *American Journal of Orthopsychiatry, 64,* 545-553.

Burke, P. (1996). *Gender shock: Exploring the myths of male and female.* New York: Doubleday.

Cass, V. C. (1979). Homosexual identity formation: A theoretical model. *Journal of Homosexuality, 4,* 219-235.

Chan, C. (1989). Issues of identity development among Asian-American lesbians and gay men. *Journal of Counseling and Development, 68*(1), 16-20.

Chauncey, G. (1994). *Gay New York: Gender, urban culture, and the making of the gay male world, 1890-1940.* New York: Basic Books.

Coleman, E. (1981.) Developmental stages of the coming out process. *The Journal of Homosexuality, 7*(2/3), 31-43.

Compas, B. E., Hinden, B. R., and Gerhardt, C. A. (1995). Adolescent development: pathways and processes of risk and resilience. *Annual Review of Psychology, 46* 265-293.

Comstock, D. G. (1991). *Violence against lesbians and gay men.* New York: Columbia University Press.

D'Augelli, A. (1989). The development of a helping community for lesbians and gay men: A case study in community psychology. *Journal of Community Psychology, 17,* 18-29.

D'Augelli, A. (1990). Community psychology and the HIV epidemic: The development of helping communities. *Journal of Community Psychology, 18,* 337-346.

D'Augelli, A. and Garnets, L. (1995). Lesbian, gay, and bisexual communities. In A. D'Augelli and C. Patterson (Eds.), *Lesbian, gay, and bisexual identities over the lifespan* (pp. 293-320). New York: Oxford University Press.

Delgado, M. and Humm-Delgado, D. (1982). Natural support systems: Sources of strength in Hispanic communities. *Social Work, 27,* 83-89.

D'Emilio, J. (1983). *Sexual politics, sexual communities: The making of a homosexual minority in the United States, 1940-1970.* Chicago: University of Chicago Press.

Duberman, M. (1991). *About time: Exploring the gay past.* New York: Meridian.

Duberman, M. (1993). *Stonewall.* New York: Dutton.

Duberman, M., Vicinus, M., and Chauncey Jr., G. (1989). *Hidden from history: Reclaiming the gay and lesbian past.* New York: Meridian.

Dulaney, D. D. and Kelly, J. J. (1982). Improving services to gay and lesbian clients. *Social Work, 27*(2), 178-183.

Espin, O. (1987). Issues of identity in the psychology of Latina lesbians. In Boston Lesbian Psychologies Collective (Ed.), *Lesbian psychologies: Explorations and challenges* (pp. 35-51). Urbana, IL: University of Illinois Press.

Faderman, L. (1991). *Old girls and twilight lovers: A history of lesbian life in twentieth-century America.* New York: Columbia University Press.

Feinberg, L. (1993). *Stone butch blues.* Ithaca, NY: Firebrand Books.

Feinberg, L. (1996). *Transgender warriors.* Boston: Beacon Press.

Germain, C. B. (1978). General-systems theory and ego psychology: An ecological perspective. *Social Service Review,* 535-550.

Germain, C. B. (1981). The ecological approach to people-environment transactions. *Social Casework: The Journal of Contemporary Social Work, 62,* 323-331.

Germain, C. B. (1985). The place of community work within an ecological approach to social work practice. In S. H. Taylor and R. W. Roberts (Eds.), *Theory and practice of community social work* (pp. 30-55). New York: Columbia University Press.

Germain, C. B. and Gitterman, A. (1996). *The life model of social work practice,* second edition. New York: Columbia University Press.

Gitterman, A. and Shulman, L. (Eds.). (1986). *The mutual aid group and the life cycle.* Itasca, IL: Peacock.

Goffman, E. (1963). *Stigma: Notes on the management of a spoiled identity.* Englewood Cliffs, NJ: Prentice-Hall.

Gutierrez, L. (1990). Working with women of color: An empowerment perspective. *Social Work, 35,* 149-153.

Gutierrez, L. and Ortega, R. (1991). Developing methods to empower Latinos: The importance of groups. *Social Work with Groups, 14*(2), 22-44.

Guttierrez, L., Alvarez, A. R., Nemon, H., and Lewis, E. A. (1996). Multicultural community organizing: A strategy for change. *Social Work, 41*(5), 501-508.

Hanson, B. (1996). The violence we face as lesbians and gay men: The landscape both outside and inside our communities. In M. Shernoff (Ed.), *Human services for gay people: Clinical and community practice* (pp. 95-114). Binghamton, NY: Harrington Park Press.

Hasenfeld, Y. and Chesler, M. (1987). Client empowerment in the human services: Personal and professional agenda. *Journal of Applied Behavioral Science, 25,* 499-521.

Hartmann. H. (1958). *Ego psychology and the problem of adaptation.* New York: International Universities Press.

Herek, G. M. (1990). The context of anti-gay violence: Notes on cultural psychological heterosexism. *Journal of Interpersonal Violence, 5*(3), 316-333.

Hunter, J. (1990). Violence against lesbian and gay male youths. *Journal of Interpersonal Violence, 5*(3), 295-300.

Icard, L. (1985-1986). Black gay men and conflicting social identities: Sexual orientation verses racial identity. *Journal of Social Work and Human Sexuality, 4*(1-2), 83-93.

Jay, K. and Young, A. (1979). *The gay report: Lesbians and gay men speak out about sexual experiences and lifestyles.* New York: Summit.

Katz, N. (Ed.). (1976). *Gay American history: Lesbians and gay men in the U.S.A.* New York: Avon Books.

Kemp, S. (1995). Practice in communities. In C. Meyer and M. A. Mattaini (Eds.), *Foundations of social work practice* (pp. 176-204). Washington, DC: NASW Press.

Kennedy, E. L. and Davis, M. (1996). Constructing an ethnohistory of the Buffalo lesbian community: Reflexivity, dialogue, and politics. In E. Lewin and W. L. Leap (Eds.), *Out in the field: Reflections of lesbian and gay anthropologists* (pp. 171-199). Urbana: University of Illinois Press.

Kramer, L. (1989). *Reports from the Holocaust: The making of an AIDS activist.* New York: St. Martin's Press.

Krieger, S. (1982). Lesbian identity and community: Recent social science literature. *Signs, 8,* 91-108.

Lee, J. (1994). *The empowerment approach to social work practice.* New York: Columbia University Press.

Lesbian and Gay Community Services Center. (1996-1997). *Lesbian and Gay Community Services Center Annual Report.* New York: Author.

Levine, C. O. (1978). Social work with transsexuals. *Social Casework, 59*(3), 167-174.

Lloyd, G. A. and Kuszelewicz, M. A. (Eds.). (1995). *HIV disease: Lesbians, gays and the social services.* Binghamton, NY: Harrington Park Press.

Lockard, D. (1985). The lesbian community: An anthropological approach. *Journal of Homosexuality, 11,* (3-4), 83-95.

Loiacano, D. K. (1989). Gay identity issues among Black Americans: Racism, homophobia, and the need for validation. *Journal of Counseling and Development, 68,* 21-25.

Marcus, E. (1992). *Making history: The struggle for gay and lesbian equal rights, 1945-1990.* New York: Harper-Collins.

Meyer, C. (1976). *Social work practice: The changing landscape.* New York: The Free Press.

Minton, H. L. and McDonald, G. J. (1984). Homosexual identity formation as a developmental process. In J. P. DeCecco and M. G. Shively (Eds.), *Origins of sexuality and homosexuality,* (pp. 91-104). Binghamton, NY: Harrington Park Press.

Paul, J. P., Hays, R. B., and Coates, T. J. (1995). The impact of the HIV epidemic on U.S. gay male communities. In A. R. D'Augelli and C. J. Patterson (Eds.), *Gay, lesbian, and bisexual identities over the lifespan* (pp. 347-397). Oxford: Oxford University Press.

Ponse B. (1980). Finding self in the lesbian community. In M. Kirkpatrick (Ed.), *Women's sexual development* (pp. 181-200). New York: Plenum.

Rich, A. (1983). Compulsory heterosexuality and lesbian existence. In A. Snitow, C. Stansell, and S. Thompson (Eds.), *Powers of desire: The politics of sexuality* (pp. 177-205). New York: Monthly Review Press.

Rivera, F. G. and Erlich, J. L. (1995). Organizing with people of color: A perspective. In J. E. Tropman, J. Erlich, and J. Rothman (Eds.), *Tactics and techniques of community intervention* (pp. 198-213). Itasca, IL: F. E. Peacock.

Rofes, E. (1996). *Reviving the tribe: Regenerating gay men's sexuality and culture in the ongoing epidemic.* Binghamton, NY: Harrington Park Press.

Russo, V. (1981). *The celluloid closet: Homosexuality in the movies.* New York: Harper and Row.

Saleebey, D. (1991). *The strengths perspective in social work practice.* New York: Longman.

Shilts, R. (1982). *The mayor of Castro Street: The life and times of Harvey Milk.* New York: St. Martin's Press.

Shilts, R. (1987). *And the band played on: People, politics, and the AIDS epidemic.* New York: St. Martin's Press.

Shilts, R. (1993). *Conduct unbecoming: Gays and lesbians in the United States military.* New York: St. Martin's Press.

Simon, B. (1994). *The empowerment tradition in American social work: A history.* New York: Columbia University Press.

Solomon, B. (1976). *Black empowerment: Social work in oppressed communities.* New York: Columbia University Press.

Staples, L. (1990). Powerful ideas about empowerment. *Administration in Social Work, 14*(2), 29-42.

Troiden, R. R. (1993). The formation of homosexual identities. In L. D. Garnets and D. G. Kimmel (Eds.), *Psychological perspectives on lesbian and gay male experiences* (pp. 191-217). New York: Columbia University Press.

Vaid, U. (1995). *Virtual equality: The mainstreaming of gay and lesbian liberation.* New York: Anchor Books.

Verghese, A. (1994). *My own country: A doctor's story of a town and its people in the age of AIDS.* New York: Simon and Schuster.

Weick, A. and Pope, L. (1988). Knowing what's best: A new look at self-determination. *Social casework,69*(1), 10-16.

Weick, A., Rapp, C., Sullivan, W. P., and Kisthardt, W. (1989). A strengths perspective of social work practice. *Social Work, 34*(4), 350-354.

Weil, M. (1986). Women, community, and organizing. In N. VanDenBergh and L. B. Cooper (Eds.), *Feminist visions for social work* (pp. 187-210). Silver Spring, MD: NASW.

Weil, M. O. (1996). Community building: Building community practice. *Social Work, 41*(5), 481-500.

Wicks, L. K. (1978). Transsexualism: A social work approach. *Health and Social Work, 2*(1), 179-193.

Chapter 11

Social Work Practice with Gay Men and Lesbians Within Organizations

George A. Appleby

The premise of this chapter is that U.S. society will reject continued attempts to defend discrimination against lesbian and gay people in the name of "family values" or "special rights" or "preservation of morale" or any other meaningless slogan. Such discrimination will be seen for what it really is: bigotry. However, social change is slow and discriminatory attitudes and behaviors will continue to be oppressive environmental and organizational influences on lesbian and gay social workers employed by human service agencies. This vestige of homophobia and heterosexism, therefore, must become the target of social work intervention (Appleby, 1995).

Sussal (1994), drawing upon the extensive research on organizational structures and their psychosocial impact, directed specific attention to the employees of social service agencies. A convincing case was made for the workplace having the potential to promote feelings of personal validation and a source of mental health. The workplace itself, however, can also become a source of emotional distress. Menzies-Lyth (1988) studied the ways the workplace can become destructive. She noted that anxieties not handled openly through discussion may result in an increased likelihood that rigid and injurious defenses against conflictual interactions may be developed. These include "prohibitions against talking about uncomfortable anxiety producing topics, unnecessarily harsh disciplinary practices, rigid lines of hierarchical relationships, and scapegoating. The impact on the individual employee in these circumstances can result in feelings of worthlessness and self-devaluation" (p. 91). She suggested that lesbians and gays are subjected to a breadth of discriminatory feedback in their daily lives that no other segment of the population must undergo. "It is not uncommon for public policies and practices to disregard lesbian and gay special needs, while at the same time not even acknowledging their existence. [This is an exercise of the most destructive defense, denial]. A conspiracy of silence exists which is anxiety producing and painful" (Sussal, 1994, pp. 90-91). While the dynamics of homophobia and heterosexism have been considered in detail elsewhere, the present discussion warrants at least an examination of some of the key correlates. Power and powerlessness are the most weighty of these correlates. Pellegrini (1992) in her study of gender inequality indicated that oppression, a key concept that ties sexism and homophobia together, is all about power: the power to enforce a particular worldview; the power to deny equal access to housing, employment opportunities, and health care; the power to alternately define and to efface difference; and the power to set the terms of power. Pharr (1988), in her examination of homophobia as a weapon of sexism, noted that some of the following are elements of all oppression: the imposition of normative behavior supported by institutional and economic power; social definition as "other"; invisibility of the "outsiders"; distortion and stereotyping; blaming the victim; and internalized oppression. Power exists on various levels: individual, interactive, as well as societal. Power is the capacity to produce desired effects on others, perceived mastery over self and others, and the capacity to influence the forces that affect one's life.

Most gay and lesbian scholars who view power and oppression from a social psychological or sociopolitical framework reference each of the above elements in their analysis of homophobia and heterosexism (Appleby and Anastas, in press; Blumenfeld, 1992; D'Emilio, 1983; Herek and Berrill, 1992). Gay men and lesbians share similar life experiences with all other oppressed people, and power or the lack thereof is central to their social functioning.

The converse of power, powerlessness is the inability to exert such influence. It is painful because the feeling of controlling one's destiny to some reasonable extent is the essential psychological component of all aspects of life. A sense of power is critical to one's mental health. Power is manifest in the individual's sense of mastery or competence.

Social work has been ambivalent about its own power or the use of power in general. Throughout the profession's literature there appears to be a reluctance to discuss professional power, as if the discussion alone might imply a collusion in the misuse of power, oppression. Social work scholars concerned with individual or societal oppression have all come to the conclusion that power is core to an understanding of person:environment as experienced by all minorities or to the development of appropriate social work interventions with these groups (Germain and Gitterman, 1996). This contemporary understanding of power is also reflected in the growing influence of "empowerment" as primary outcome and process in practice theory.

Social work has had a long and proud tradition of advocating on behalf of vulnerable and oppressed people—that is, accessing power for others—and lesbian and gay clients have not been exceptions. Self-advocacy, unfortunately, has too often been interpreted by some social workers in the past as crass self-interest, and thus less worthy of attention. In recent years, with the advent of union organizing and legislative lobbying around professional licensing and standards, third-partying payment, and managed care policies, this trend is being reversed. It is the position taken in this essay that all social workers, especially minorities, and specifically lesbian or gay social workers must begin to reframe self-advocacy as a matter of gaining personal and societal power in the areas of civil rights, organizational (agency) recognition and equity, and mental health in the workplace. It will be argued that the profession's self-advocacy is mandated by the code of ethics, that it is supported by organizational and political realities, and that it is consistent with contemporary practice perspectives and skills. The case will be made that lesbian and gay social workers should begin to focus on their own workplace to create an inclusive, productive environment for everyone. Finally, it will be argued that lesbian and gay social workers should form coalitions with other minorities and like-minded people to press for a specific strategy of "diversity management" that is both inclusive and clearly stated in terms of outcomes that are tied to professional productivity.

CODE OF ETHICS

The National Association of Social Workers (NASW) joined the American Psychological Association and the American Psychiatric Association in the 1970s to challenge the indefensible position that homosexuality is a mental illness resulting from pathological development. The mental health professions came to this position after an extensive review of the existing research and the clinical experiences of its members. Each profession now views homosexuality not as an illness but as another path to psychosocial adaptation. In 1979, the social work profession included nondiscrimination language based on sexual orientation in its newly developed Code of Ethics. The code is based on the fundamental values of the social work profession that include the worth, dignity, and uniqueness of all persons as well as the advancement of their rights and opportunities. It is also based on the nature of social work, which fosters conditions that promote these values as ingredients of optimal social functioning. The code offers general principles to guide conduct in situations that have ethical implications. Specifically, social workers shall not "practice, condone, facilitate or collaborate with any form of discrimination on the basis of race, color, sex, sexual orientation . . . (National Association of Social Workers *Code of Ethics*, Section II., F., 3., 1993). The individual social worker and agency are expected to deliver appropriate and nondiscriminatory services to all clients. While this language is specific to the worker's ethical responsibility to clients, it can be logically generalized to his or her ethical responsibility to colleagues because of the code's emphasis on respect, courtesy, fairness, and good faith. General language is again introduced in reference to employers and employing organizations: " . . . to improve the employing agency's policies and procedures . . . (IV., L., 1.) . . . act to prevent and eliminate discrimination in the employing organization's work assignments and in its employment policies and practices" (IV., L., 3., 1993). Finally, restated in the code in relation to ethical responsibility to society is the same language: "The social worker should act to prevent and eliminate discrimination against any person or group on the basis of . . . sexual orientation . . . " (VI., P., 1., 1993). The revised code, adopted by the 1996 Delegate Assembly and enacted in 1997, is a clearer articulation of the profession's values of service, social justice, dignity and worth of the person, importance of human relationships, integrity, and competence. The language related to sexual orientation is as emphatic as the original document. The code goes well beyond advocacy on behalf of clients, to mandate self-advocacy as a means of ending discrimination against lesbian and gay social workers in social agencies and professional organizations (Code of Ethics Revision Committee, August 7, 1996). While most agencies are effective in the application of the code to clients, some have yet to move beyond cultural homophobia in relation to policies governing the workplace. The code, then, has the potential to be one of the most powerful tools in support of ending bigotry and agency-based discrimination.

Initially, NASW adopted an educational strategy to advance the code. Eventually, the association formed state and national committees on inquiry (COI) to adjudicate violations of the code. The code and the related adjudication procedures are powerful instruments of social justice for lesbians and gay men, holding both the practitioner and the social agency accountable. Violation of the code may bring public censure that could result in public humiliation and possible loss of funds and accreditation status for an agency and loss of employment for the individual. Most COI cases related to sexual orientation focused on client discrimination and seldom on agency-based worker discrimination. For those social workers whose work world negates their personhood and denies their unique needs, self-advocacy apparently has not become the norm.

ORGANIZATIONAL AND POLITICAL REALITIES

In recent years, NASW has taken on an advocacy role in relation to expanding civil rights of this still-marginalized group. Social policy now reflects an appreciation that gay and lesbian discrimination is a violation of both the right of privacy and equal protection under the law as guaranteed by the U.S. Constitution and the Bill of Rights. These are the basic rights of citizenship. The Constitution does not allow for exceptions. This change from an educational focus on the mental health consequences to an emphasis on civil rights has not been an easy task. Nonjudgmental attitudes are necessary to support social change and to end individual and organizational prejudice. Homophobia and heterosexism are social forces that permeate all aspects of social life; social service agencies and social work professionals are not immune. Attitudes about homosexuality in the helping professions as a whole have been changing markedly since the 1970s. Unfortunately, both workers and clients may still be affected by the residue of outmoded psychological theory that until recently viewed homosexuality as pathology. Scholars warn that the worker's feelings, attitudes, and level of comfort with gay or lesbian orientation must be examined; they require self-exploration over time. Studies continue to suggest that negative attitudes toward homosexuality and homosexual clients persist among some social workers and social work students (DeCrescenzo, 1984; Greene, 1994; Harris, Nightingale, and Owen, 1995; Eliason, 1995). Prejudice toward lesbian, gay, and bisexual social workers results in discriminatory personnel practices and unnecessary stress.

In 1977, the Delegate Assembly of the NASW approved a policy statement on gay issues, affirming the association's understanding of the social, economic, political, and mental health consequences of discrimination and prejudice, and thus outlined a modest action plan focusing on the education of the profession.. The following year, the NASW Board of Directors established its first Task Force on Gay Issues to help carry out the earlier mandate. In 1979, the task force was restructured as an authorized committee of the association and in 1982 it was renamed the National Committee on Lesbian and Gay Issues (NCOLGI) with resources to advance the education of membership. The committee supported the development of a monograph, *Lesbian and Gay Issues: A Resource Manual for Social Workers* (Hidalgo, Peterson, and Woodman, 1985); encouraged NASW Press to solicit articles related to lesbian and gay issues; and identified relevant workshops for the annual conference. Throughout this period, the energy of the committee and thus the association was directed toward mounting a response to the AIDS pandemic, and to a lesser extent, educating membership about gay and lesbian issues. In 1993, the committee became a bylaws-mandated equity unit, along with the National Committee on Women's Issues (NCOWI) and the National Committee on Minority Affairs (NCOMA), each accountable to the board. It took ten years, 1977 to 1987, after the first social policy statement was adopted, for the Delegate Assembly to revise significantly the original document and to rename it *Lesbian and Gay Issues*. Monumental change took place in 1996 when the Delegate Assembly approved a bylaws amendment that added sexual orientation to its list of protected classes in the association's affirmative action plan. Along with this change which places the profession in the forefront of its sister disciplines, a major revision of its 1987 policy statement was adopted. This latest statement, *Lesbian, Gay, and Bisexual Issues* (National Association of Social Workers, 1996), is probably the most progressive position taken by any of the legal, educational, health, human service, and mental health professional associations:

> It is the position of NASW that same-gender sexual orientation should be afforded the same respect and rights as opposite-gender orientation. NASW asserts that discrimination and prejudice directed against any group are damaging to the social, emotional, and economic well-being of the affected group and of society as a whole. NASW is committed to advancing policies and practices that will improve the status and well-being of all lesbian, gay and bisexual people.

> NASW believes that nonjudgmental attitudes toward sexual orientation allow social workers to offer optimal support and services to lesbian, gay, and bisexual people. The profession supports and empowers lesbian, gay, and bisexual people through all phases of the coming out process and beyond. The profession believes discriminatory statutes, policies, and actions that diminish the quality of life for lesbian, gay, and bisexual people and that force many to live their lives in secrecy should be prevented and eliminated. NASW supports the right of the individual to self-disclosed sexual orientation. NASW encourages the development of supportive practice environments for lesbian, gay, and bisexual clients and colleagues. . . . The rights and well-being of the children of lesbian, gay, and bisexual people should be an integral part of all these considerations.

NASW affirms its commitment to work toward full social and legal acceptance and recognition of lesbian, gay, and bisexual people. . . . To this end, NASW supports legislation, regulation, policies, judicial review, political action, and changes in social work policy statements and the NASW Code of Ethics and any other means necessary to establish and protect the equal rights of all people without regard to sexual orientation. NASW is committed to working toward the elimination of prejudice and discrimination both inside and outside the profession. (NASW, 1996, pp. 2-3)

At this same Delegate Assembly, approval was given to policy statements and resolutions related to full representation at all levels of leadership and employment, the broadening of nondiscrimination statements to include sexual orientation in all social agencies, universities, professional associations, and funding organizations; to exact the association to campaign against any laws allowing discriminatory practices in immigration, employment, housing, professional credentialing, licensing, public accommodation, child custody and the right to marry; and to oppose exclusion from the military and other forms of government services. "All social work practitioners, administrators, and educators are encouraged to take action to ensure that the dignity and rights of lesbian, gay and bisexual employees, clients and students are upheld and that these rights are codified in agency policies" (NASW, 1996, pp. 5-6). Policy became more than an abstraction when in 1996 the NASW Board of Directors charged the National Committee on Lesbian, Gay, and Bisexual Issues to go beyond education to achieve its purpose: "to further the cause of social justice by promoting and defending the rights of persons suffering injustices and oppression because they are lesbian, gay, or bisexual" (National Association of Social Workers National Committee on Lesbian, Gay, and Bisexual Issues, June 1996). The committee has been charged to address policy development and practice standards; to engage in civil rights activities and advocacy; to continue pressing for professional education; and to assist the association in its own organizational development in relation to gay, lesbian, and bisexual rights and privileges. The corporate political and organizational will has been clearly stated.

This, then, is another powerful resource for practitioners committed to changing the climate of social agencies.

CONTEMPORARY PRACTICE

Social work is an agency-based profession with well-recognized organizational skills in service delivery and formal and informal resources management. These skills evolved over the last hundred years as the profession matured within its organizational context. Today, this knowledge, and these skills and processes have become the core of all social work practice, commonly referred to as generalist or foundation practice. The emphasis of this section is the environmental focus of practice, the goal of empowerment, and the organizational skills of self-advocacy.

The generalist social worker possesses an integrated view of people and environments and uses appropriate interventions to empower consumers at all social system levels. Nurturing environments have been given much more theoretical attention with the introduction of Germain and Gitterman (1980) and Germain's (1991) advancement of the ecological perspective. Much of the empirical work in this area has sought to understand various client environments and to reassess the effectiveness of social work interventions. Scholars focusing on either clinical or generalist approaches to practice have drawn heavily on the ecological metaphor.

Another theme of contemporary practice is empowerment. Empowerment may be defined as the enabling of a client population to handle problems on its own, with the feeling of a growing capacity to take their lives into their own hands. Gutierrez (1990) defines empowerment as "a process of increasing personal, interpersonal, or political power so that individuals can take action to improve their situation . . . "; it is the "development of increased power or control." It is a process necessary to cope in a hostile world and may mean (1) increasing self-efficacy; (2) developing a sense of mastery, initiative, and action; and (3) fostering group consciousness and a "sense of shared fate." This facilitates a person's ability for reducing self-blame and seeing many problems as being collective rather than just their's alone. Problems are often a function of societal power arrangements. Self-blame is often responsible for feelings of depression and immobilization. When people feel competent and self-assured, they are more capable of assuming personal responsibility for change (Morales, 1995). The shades of mental health theory and practice run through these discussions of empowerment.

In relation to lesbian and gay social work, Sussal (1994) reminded us that the workplace provides a unique situation in which an environment supportive of mental health can be structured by influencing and setting policies that obviate discrimination, developing programs to raise consciousness about gay and lesbian issues, and delivering direct services to gays and lesbians and their family members or co-workers.

Generalists regard clients in relation to the social milieu, view problems in the context of the situation, and seek solutions within both personal and environmental structures. Many of the empowering processes, as well as the functions of generalist social work entail some degree of organizational sophistication. Many scholars studied the array of professional and client roles in relation to organizational processes associated with client and worker's tasks, e.g., accessing, processing, utilizing, and communicating information. McPheeters (1971), Teare and McPheeters (1970, 1982), Pincus and Minahan (1976), and Johnson (1995) analyzed helping roles while Siporin (1975) analyzed role models and Compton and Galaway (1994) and Connaway and Gentry (1988) studied role sets and interventive roles. DuBois and Miley (1996) extend this scholarship by identifying the organizational nature of practice implicit in the core roles and functions of generalist practice. The role of consultant (for problem solving) includes activities directed toward empowering clients to resolve problems, fostering organizational development, coordinating program and policy development, and mentoring. A second role, resource manager, includes activities commonly thought as brokering, convening, and mediating. The third role, educator, covers a range of teaching and training activities aimed at clients, colleagues, and the public.

One specific skill continually referenced by each of the scholars mentioned is advocacy. In situations where adequate services do not exist or are not accessible, the social worker assumes an advocacy function. As an advocate, he or she is concerned with making the social welfare system responsive to the unmet needs of the client. According to Briar (1968), the social worker as advocate is the client's supporter, advisor, champion, and if need be, representative in his or her dealings with the court, the police, the social agency, and other organizations that affect the client's well-being. Advocacy, then, is an organizational skill. Because of the currency of this skill, social workers understand the pervasiveness and extensiveness of organizations in our national life, and that organizations determine what and how resources are to be distributed to both consumers of our services and to those of us who provide the service. They determine the direction (or what appears to be nondirection) of the society. Also, they are barriers to social change and social justice, just as they are the very basis of change and the guarantor of the benefits of social justice.

Social workers have come belatedly to appreciate the unique organizational dynamics of agency-based practice, with its own well-developed theoretical base (organizational theory) and its range of macro intervention skills, which are similar and unlike those of clinical or interpersonal practice. Inappropriately, practitioners tend to draw upon interpersonal and developmental theory and, too often, upon a family systems metaphor when analyzing organizational behavior. This is akin to explaining soil erosion as the result of the land's weakened immunologic reaction to ozone depletion in the stratosphere. Interventions also tend to be more interpersonal than task group or administrative. A composite view of organizations that blends content from sociology, psychology, economics, management, anthropology, political science, and industrial relations should inform assessment at this level. The point is worth emphasizing that this is an important body of theory to inform practice designed to empower lesbian, gay, and bisexual clients, as well as employees in their pursuit of a nondiscriminatory workplace environment.

What, then, from this body of practice knowledge, theory, and research, helps us to understand the unique reality of lesbians and gays within human service organizations and directs energy toward the improvement of that reality? Theory suggests that organizations tend to grow. Growth is equated with success. Even in a no-growth economy, public and private organizations try to grow at one another's expense. In addition to their growth in size, another important consideration gives contemporary organizations an unprecedented role in contemporary society: the modern organization is a *legal* entity, just like the individual (Coleman, 1974). The legality is granted by the state, itself a legal creation. While the individual is given a set of rights and responsibilities by the state, these same rights and responsibilities are extended to organizations. These rights, coupled with size, give organizations an enormous amount of power within the state. The state or government is more comfortable dealing with other organizations than with individual persons, and thus tends to provide more preferential treatment in terms of taxation or rights to privacy.

Hall (1977) in his classic summary of organizational theory, pointed out that government organizations receive power through mandates from the legislature and will seek to maintain that power even if no purpose is being served. In other words, organizations grow, maintain themselves, and continue their operations regardless of the motivations of their members. Organizations process information and to accomplish this end they structure themselves by establishing roles, lines of communication, and ranks in organization. Procedures are established in advance to deal with most possible events. These structures virtually force certain things to be communicated and suppress other things. Individuals who process and interpret the information that is passed on to people in decision-making position have influence or power. Professionally, social workers have come to respect the inexorable power of organizations and have used this power to expand the health, mental health and human service rights and benefits of clients. Thus, following an understanding of organizational theory and the professional experience with the manipulation of power, the strategy should then be to change the agency's environment with the goal of increasing the power of lesbian and gay workers as they coalesce with other devalued constituencies.

STRATEGIES FOR AN INCLUSIVE WORKPLACE

Those charged with the management of any organization do not typically address a problem until two things happen. First, they become reasonably sure that a problem exists, and second, they become convinced that trying to solve the problem will be good for agency growth and survival. Winfeld and Spielman (1995) suggested that public and private organizations are attempting to adapt to the changing demographics of both their clients/consumers and their employees. The vogue strategy is diversity management, which is now viewed more as a core administrative issue and less as strictly a human resources issue. The distinction is a crucial one. Although administrators have not doubted that proper management and support programs are important, those programs have not been tied into performance outcomes. Some vague relationship between caring for staff and their resulting performance has always been acknowledged, but it was never considered an empirical cause and effect. That is changing in industry and in some sectors of the public arena. If the point of a diversity management effort is to create a harassment-free, satisfactory, cooperative, productive, and profitable/effective workplace for all, then it must include sexual orientation as a diversity factor.

The business and industrial relations literature offers evidence that companies with progressive, people-oriented strategies experience better results in terms of customer satisfaction, profitability, and global competitiveness (Lyndenberg, Marlin, and Strub, 1986). While the terms may be different, the underlying concepts are relevant to the environment both in and outside a social agency. A progressive company or social service organization benefits from the ability to take full advantage of the skills and knowledge of all of its employees. A big part of this benefit is felt in allowing each person to perform to his or her greatest potential, unfettered by fear of prejudice; but it is demonstrated in another way as well. Members of a given group often understand the customs, practices, and requirement of that group better than people who are not members. Therefore, tapping into the cultural expertise and knowledge of certain employee constituencies can pay rich dividends in new and relevant services.

Another significant factor is the very real issue of productivity. Work is a task, but it is also a social activity. People need and expect to be able to express themselves to the fullest, and when they can't, they are unhappy. That unhappiness may eventually sabotage the efforts of the work group and by extension weaken the performance of the whole organization.

There are other reasons to include lesbian and gay employees into an overall diversity strategy: law, service effectiveness, and common sense. The legal landscape in relation to gay rights changes continually. As of this writing, gay rights are not protected by the U.S. Constitution. No federal job protection exits in this country. The Employment Non-Discrimination Act (ENDA), which would provide such protection, has yet to be passed by Congress. Nine states—California, Connecticut, Hawaii, Massachusetts, Minnesota, New Jersey, Rhode Island, Vermont, and Wisconsin, and the District of Columbia—offer full civil rights legal protection to gay people. Between fifteen and eighteen others cover some degree of protection with very tenuous executive orders. Approximately one hundred and sixty-five cities and counties have ordinances that do not carry the weight of law (National Gay and Lesbian Task Force, Policy Institute, 1996). While these laws and ordinances vary in power, each represents a building block upon which precedents are being set. Many of these precedents have implications for employers. Agencies that operate in a state, city, or county with a sexual orientation nondiscrimination law or order are in violation of the law if it does not include sexual orientation as a protected characteristic in its written nondiscrimination policy. Violators can be sued or brought before the state's human rights commission.

Organizations can expect more of their gay employees to insist upon discrimination protection and equitable benefits in the workplace. And those organizations would do well to listen. The reason is simple. In those places where the law does not protect and provide for inclusion of sexual minorities, gay people work under enormous strain. They cannot perform at their best under these oppressive circumstances. In many cases discrimination is unlawful; it is always unproductive and unprofitable (Winfeld and Spielman, 1995, p. 11).

Effectiveness is another reason for organizations to take a proactive stance. The experience of industry suggests that adopting discriminatory policies is detrimental to economic health. Human rights are never far divorced from economics. According to a 1996 *Newsweek* poll, nearly 84 percent of Americans support equal employment rights for gay men and lesbians. The Human Rights Campaign found that in 1994, 70 percent the voting population did not realize that antigay job discrimination is still widespread and predominantly legal (Goldberg, 1996). Organizations that support gay and lesbian employees and their requirements will be rewarded, and those that resist inclusion will see the results in their annual reports, decreased service caseloads, and funding sources.

Common sense is perhaps the most compelling reason for including gay and lesbian workers in the agency's diversity mix. They are already there. About 10 percent of the population is believed to be gay or lesbian, yet a much higher but unconfirmed percentage is estimated for the health and social services workforce. About 21 million (conservative estimate) lesbians and gay men live and work in the United States alone. Some studies estimate that they are the single largest minority in the workforce (Williamson, 1993). They need and want the quite ordinary freedom of visibility without reprisals.

Winfeld and Spielman (1995) in their analysis of human diversity in private industry sum up by observing that all organizations have it within their power to a take an affirming position on nondiscrimination and to proactively ensure that all members understand the dynamics of the nondiscrimination policy. The reason is simple: Unless organizations take a proactive stance, they can be sure that they will lose customers/clients and talented employees to competitors who have. Inclusion is a very small price to pay for effectiveness and productivity. It must be acknowledged that some agencies, either through religious conviction or homophobia or both, are hesitant or want to avoid this subject altogether. Some fear that they will lose clients or community support if they take an ethical/legal stance. They are afraid that having an inclusive policy will be interpreted as giving tacit approval, and that clients who hold the opposite view will seek services elsewhere. This argument would have little merit if the discussion were to focus on racism or sexism, but because homophobia is so institutionalized, this contradiction is seldom raised. Leaving the ethics of this situation aside, the answer is simple: Acknowledgment of and education about something does not equal endorsement of it. Providing for the concerns of a particular constituency in the agency does not mean that you endorse the members of that constituency, their behavior, or their beliefs. It is quite pragmatic, in that it simply signals that the agency is committed to all its employees with no exceptions.

The agency can do many things to secure and maintain the best effort of its employees. In return for equitable benefits, programs, and policies, the employer has the right to expect dedication, loyalty, self-motivation, and cooperation from all employees at all times. From a gay and lesbian perspective, the trade is a simple one, the same as is expected by and granted to heterosexual employees: a safe working environment, equitable benefits, and appropriate public support (Winfeld and Spielman, 1996).

A safe work environment is demonstrated and encouraged by three things: (1) a nondiscrimination policy that expressly includes sexual orientation; (2) diversity education that includes a comprehensive module on sexual orientation and; (3) equitable human resource policies, and the support of a gay/straight employees alliance. Equitable benefits means providing to the partners of lesbian and gay employees the same benefits, including health coverage, that are accorded the families of other employees—in essence, equal pay for equal work.

Equitable benefit plans may include hard benefits, such as medical and dental care, and soft benefits, such as adoption benefits, bereavement and family leave policies, employee assistance programs, parenting leave, use of health and fitness programs, relocation policy, and sick leave. While these benefits are commonly available in the private sector, access to school records, visitation in hospitals and prisons, and home purchase loans are usually offered by the public sector. Other areas in which agencies can take a proactive stance toward equity are agency-paid pension plans and benefits under COBRA and the Family and Medical Leave Act of 1993.

The law and justice are not the same thing, but the terms are frequently used interchangeably. While there are few direct legal precedents for domestic partner benefits, there are ample precedents of justice. Both as matters of justice and law, an employer is obligated to provide equal pay for equal work to its employees. By providing benefits to the families of married employees and denying the same to families of unmarried employees, the employer is violating that obligation and discriminating according to the marital status and sexual orientation of its employees. By refusing to provide the same benefits to unmarried employees as it provides to married employees, the employer may be violating any number of previously mentioned city, county, and state laws.

COMING OUT AT THE WORKPLACE

Gays and lesbians are different from visibly recognizable minorities because they must decide whether to come out whenever meeting someone new or every time a personal topic comes up at work. If they stay in the closet, they may cope by not telling the whole story or by simply avoiding personal conversations. This takes a lot of energy. The stress of not being open either to oneself or to coworkers is taxing. Lesbians and gay men and their heterosexual allies who deal every day with the silence and intolerance of their agencies or organizations deserve a lot of affirming messages. They need to hear that they are not shameful and that even the smallest details of their lives that reflect their sexual orientation are worthy of having someone hear them (Zuckerman and Simons, 1996). The growing literature on lesbians and gays in the workplace (see Ellis and Riggle, 1996) suggests that the most effective weapon against homophobia is for gay and lesbian social work employees to come out. This action will counter stereotypes and end the isolation and the institutional process of blaming the victim as they present themselves publicly as competent, functioning, visible representatives of their community (Pharr, 1988).

While coming out appears to be most effective, there are several other steps that can be taken in response to questionable personnel practice: file an objection and if that does not work, bring legal suit against overt discrimination. It is important to remember that coming out is a painful and liberating process involving complex decisions under the best circumstances, but when it pertains to the workplace, it is affected by the socioeconomic climate, perceived job risk, prior loss of job due to coming out, income, child-related work, gender structure of the workplace, as well as religion and self-hate (Schneider, 1986) . Social workers must respect that while coming out will promote self-esteem and renewed energy with the removal of significant psychological and social barriers, it also entails risks and courage and timing.

SELF-ADVOCACY REVISITED

It is too easy to overestimate the climate of acceptance. Collective action is more effective than individually playing Don Quixote fighting windmills. The process of building the support of other minorities and like-minded allies will prove more fruitful. Gay men, lesbians, and heterosexuals have been working together successfully since the beginning of time. What is different today is that many people now openly live out their sexual orientation. This challenges straight and gay people alike to deal with their fears and prejudices on the job so that all can be creative and productive together.

The following steps are recommended in the process of assisting agencies to become nurturing environments that champion the civil rights and the well-being of lesbian and gay employees: (1) start with an educational program related to sexual orientation for all employees, (2) follow this up with supportive programs that offer mentoring by someone with organizational status, or arrange an opportunity to work with a coming-out coach who has had a successful experience, and finally, programs that encourage joining support groups and networks of lesbians, gay men, and their allies. Understandably, such a network might become the constituency group, the medium for self-advocacy, most invested in pressing for a safe work environment, equitable benefits, and appropriate public support.

RESOURCES

- WorkNet (an advocacy organization based in Washington, DC) has been amassing information aimed at persuading Congress to pass the Employment Non-Discrimination Act (ENDA). It also shares the tools necessary to lobby for fairness at work and information on employers with nondiscrimination policies, domestic partnership policies, and employee support groups.

A referral service is available for workers who need legal assistance regarding job discrimination. WorkNet can be reached on the Human Rights Campaign (HRC) Website-http://www.hrcusa.org or by calling 202-628-4160.

- National Committee on Lesbian, Gay, and Bisexual Issues of the National Association of Social Workers. Contact: Luisa Lopez or Indra Malani, NASW, 750 First Street, NE, Suite 700, Washington, DC 20002-4341, call 202-408-8600.
- American Civil Liberties Union–Gay and Lesbian Rights Project. 132 West 43rd St., New York, NY 10036, call 212-807-1700.
- Human Rights Campaign. 1101 14th Street, NW, Suite 200, Washington, DC 20005, call 202-628-4160.
- Lambda Legal Defense and Education Fund. 666 Broadway, 12th Floor, New York, NY 10012, call 212-995-8585.
- National Gay and Lesbian Task Force–Workplace Project. 2320 17th Street, NW, Washington, DC 20009, call 202-332-6483 x3361.

REFERENCES

Appleby, G. A. (1995). AIDS and homophobia/heterosexism. In G. A. Lloyd and M. A. Kuszelewicz (Eds.), *HIV disease: Lesbians, gays and the social services* (pp. 1-24). Binghamton, NY: Harrington Park Press.

Appleby, G. A. and Anastas, J. (in press). *Not just a passing phase: Social work with lesbian, gay and bisexual people.* New York: Columbia University Press.

Blumenfeld, W. J. (Ed.) (1992). *Homophobia: How we all pay the price.* Boston: Beacon Press.

Briar, S. (1968). The casework predicament, *Social Work, 13*(1), 5-11.

Code of Ethics Revision Committee. (August 7, 1996) Memorandum: Code of ethics revised draft. Washington, DC: National Association of Social Workers.

Coleman, J. S. (1974) *Power and the structure of society.* New York: W.W. Norton and Company.

Compton, B. and Galaway, B. (1994). *Social work processes,* fifth edition. Pacific Grove, CA: Brooks/Cole Publishing Company.

Connaway, R. and Gentry, M. (1988). *Social work practice.* Englewood Cliffs, NJ: Prentice Hall.

DeCrescenzo, T. A. (1984). Homophobia: A study of the attitudes of mental health professionals toward homosexuality, *Journal of Social Work and Human Sexuality, 2,* 115-136.

D'Emilio, J. (1983). *Sexual politics, sexual communities: The making of a homosexual minority in the United States; 1940-1970.* Chicago: University of Chicago Press.

DuBois, B. and Miley, K. K. (1996). *Social work: An empowering profession,* second edition. Boston: Allyn and Bacon.

Eliason, M. J. (1995). Attitudes about lesbians and gay men: A review and implications for social service training, *Journal of Gay & Lesbian Social Services,* 2(2), 73-90.

Ellis, A. L. and Riggle, E. D. B. (Eds.). (1996). Sexual identity on the job: Issues and services. [Special Issue]. *Journal of Gay & Lesbian Social Services,* 4(4).

Germain, C. B. (1991). *Human behavior and the social environment: An ecological view.* New York: Columbia University Press.

Germain, C. B. and Gitterman, A. (1980). *The life model of social work practice.* New York: Columbia University Press.

Germain, C. B. and Gitterman, A. (1996). *The life model of social work practice,* second edition. New York: Columbia University Press.

Goldberg, S. B. (1996). No special rights: Supreme court's amendment 2 decision has long-range implications, *HRC Quarterly,* (Summer), 4-5.

Greene, R. R. (1994). Social work practice within a diversity framework. In R. R. Greene (Ed.), *Human behavior theory: A diversity framework* (pp. 1-18). New York: Aldine de Gruyter.

Gutierrez, L. (1990). Working with women of color: An empowerment perspective. *Social Work,* 35(2), 149-152.

Hall, R. H. (1977). *Organizations: Structure and process,* second edition. Englewood Cliffs, NJ: Prentice-Hall, Inc.

Harris, M. B., Nightengale, J., and Owen, N. (1995). Health care professionals' experience, knowledge, and attitudes concerning homosexuality. *Journal of Gay & Lesbian Social Services,* 2(2), 91-108.

Herek, G. and Berrill, K. (1992). *Hate crimes: Confronting violence against lesbians and gay men.* Newbury Park, CA: Sage Publications.

Hidalgo, H., Peterson, T. L., and Woodman, N. J. (Eds.). (1985). *Lesbian and gay issues: A resource manual for social workers.* Washington, DC: NASW Press.

Johnson, L. C. (1995). *Social work practice: A generalist approach,* fourth edition. Boston: Allyn and Bacon.

Lyndenberg, S., Marlin, A. T., and Strub, S. O. (1986). *Rating America's corporate conscience: A proactive guide to the companies behind the products you buy.* New York: Addison-Wesley.

McPheeters, H. L. (1971). *A core of competence for baccalaureate social welfare.* Atlanta: The Undergraduate Social Welfare Manpower Project.

Menzies-Lyth, I. (1988). *Containing anxiety is social institutions: Selected essays.* London: Free Association Press.

Morales, J. (1995). Gay Latinos and AIDS: A framework for HIV/AIDS prevention education. *Journal of Gay & Lesbian Social Services,* 2(3/4), 89-105.

National Association of Social Workers. (1993). *Code of ethics.* Washington, DC: author.

National Association of Social Workers. (1996). Lesbian, gay and bisexual issues (Revised Social Policy Statement). Washington, DC: author.

National Association of Social Workers National Committee on Lesbian, Gay, and Bisexual Issues (NCOLGABI). (June 1996). Board of Directors' Committee Charge. Washington, DC: author.

National Gay and Lesbian Task Force, Policy Institute. (January 1996). Beyond the beltway: State of the states 1995. Washington, DC: author.

Pellegrini, A. (1992). S(h)ifting the terms of hetero/sexism: Gender, power, homophobia, In W. J. Blumenfeld (Ed.), *Homophobia: How we all pay the price* (pp. 39-56). Boston: Beacon Press.

Pharr, S. (1988). *Homophobia: A weapon of sexism.* Arizona: Chardon Press

Pincus, A. and Minahan, A. (1976). *Social work practice model and method.* Itasca, IL: Peacock Publishers.

Schneider, B. E. (1986). Coming out at the workplace: Bridging the private/public gap. *Journal of Work with Groups, 8*(3), 71-79.

Siporin, M. (1975). *Introduction to social work practice.* New York: Macmillan Publishing Co.

Sussal, C. M. (1994). Empowering gays and lesbians in the workplace. *Journal of Gay & Lesbian Social Services, 1*(1), 89-103.

Teare, R. J. and McPheeters, H. L. (1970). *Manpower utilization in social welfare: A report based on a symposium on manpower utilization in social welfare services.* Atlanta: Southern Regional Educational Board.

Teare, R. J. and McPheeters, H. L. (1982). A framework for practice is social welfare: Objectives and roles. In D. S. Sanders, O. Durren, and J. Fischer (Eds.), *Fundamentals of social work practice* (pp.56-72). Belmont, CA: Wadsworth Publishing Company.

Williamson, A. D. (1993). Is this the right time to come out? *Harvard Business Review,* (July/August), 26-34.

Winfeld, L. and Spielman, S. (1995). *Straight talk about gays in the workplace: Creating an inclusive, productive environment for everyone in your organization.* New York: AMACOM.

Winfeld, L. and Spielman, S. (1996). The workplace is a happening place, *HRC Quarterly,* (Summer), 12-13.

Zuckerman, A. J. and Simons, G. F. (1996). *Sexual orientation in the workplace.* Thousand Oaks: Sage Publications.

Appendix

Definitions of Key Terms

Gerald P. Mallon

Several of these definitions are based on those proposed by Schneider (1988).

The glossary is intended to orient the reader to the more commonly used vocabulary in lesbian and gay literature and speech. Language is often a source of confusion and misinformation and as such, it is important that service providers have accurate definitions. Heterosexually oriented care providers are often unfamiliar and uncomfortable with the vernacular of the gay and lesbian culture. it should be recognized that as with any subculture—particularly oppressed groups—there is a constantly changing argot. Usage may vary with generation, geographic region of the country, socioeconomic status, or cultural background.

Sex: The biological status as a female or male.

Sexual Identity: An individual's sense of self as male or female from the social and psychological perspective. Identity is the culturally informed process of expressing desires in a social role and with socially shared cultural practices within a social context.

Gender Role: The characteristics of an individual that are culturally defined as masculine or feminine.

Sexual Orientation: The commonly accepted, scientific term for the direction of sexual attraction, emotional and/or physical attraction, and its expression. Examples of sexual orientation are heterosexuality, homosexuality, and bisexuality.

Usage: The term sexual preference is habitually used to express the meaning of sexual orientation. However, sexual preference is also misinterpreted to mean that sexual attraction, including same-gender attraction, is generally a matter of conscious choice. Although such a choice might be possible (particularly for women), current research indicates that sexual orientation is not a matter of choice. Sexual orientation is, therefore, the more accurate term. Sexual preference, sexual proclivity, sexual tendencies, or the notion of turning gay or lesbian by choice are inaccurate characterizations.

Kinsey Scale: A seven-point continuum (0-6) developed by Alfred Kinsey and his associates in 1948 to describe sexual orientation. The scale ranges from 0, which denotes exclusive heterosexuality, to 6, which denotes exclusive homosexuality, with all possible gradations in between. Incorporating one's behavior, affectional preferences, fantasy, and "sense of goodness of fit," most people are located somewhere between the two extremes.

Heterosexuality: A male or female person whose sexual attraction, both physical and affectional, are primarily directed toward persons of the opposite gender.

Homosexuality: A male or female person whose sexual attraction, both physical and affectional, is primarily directed toward persons of the same gender. Other terms used to describe persons of this sexual orientation include gay and lesbian.

Bisexuality: A male or female person whose sexual attraction, both physical and affectional, is directed toward persons of both genders. Many persons who are beginning the coming our process will identify as bisexual before identifying as gay or lesbian because historically bisexuality represents a meditating position between homosexual and heterosexual in the traditional American cultural system.

Usage: Except for strictly scientific or scholarly uses, it is inappropriate to apply the terms heterosexual, homosexual, and bisexual to people. Incorrectly used these terms can be taken to indicate that sexual orientation is the sole basis of personal or group identity.

For example, a homosexual person may have ethic, gender, geographical, political, professional, and religious identities, in addition to his or her sexual identity. The term homosexual has been popularly misinterpreted as applying only to men, and is also inappropriate because of its formal, clinical tone. Therefore, it is generally advisable to use when possible the terms gay and/or lesbian to refer to people of homosexual orientation.

Sexual Minority: A group term used to identify a person who self-identifies as homosexual, gay, lesbian, bisexual, transgender, or transvestite. While it is true that all gay and lesbian persons are members of a sexual minority, not all sexual minority persons are gay.

Gay: A person whose homosexual orientation is self-defined, affirmed, or acknowledged as such. Gay also refers to homosexually oriented ideas (e.g., styles, lifestyles, literature, or values). It is believed that this term originated as a kind of code among homosexual men and women. It is a popular alternative to homosexual primarily because it is a word that comes from the gay and lesbian community. It is a way for homosexuals to communicate among and about themselves with pride.

Lesbian: A woman whose homosexual orientation is self-defined, affirmed, or acknowledged as such. Lesbian also refers to female homosexually oriented (and can refer to women-oriented) ideas, communities, or varieties of cultural expression (e.g., styles, lifestyles, literature, or values).

The term lesbian or gay usually indicates a personal or social identity, normally suggesting that the person has identified herself or himself as lesbian or gay or that a group accepts or affirms the identification. The terms are not necessarily synonymous with homosexual in that a person can be homosexual or have engaged in same-gendered activities without necessarily identifying as lesbian or gay. These latter terms have cultural, political, and social connotations in addition to sexual ones. A lesbian or gay person sees herself or himself as homosexually oriented among other sources of identity. The term lesbian historically refers to the island of Lesbos where a noted poet, Sappho, and her female followers lived in the sixth century BC.

Usage: As indicated, the term gay can refer to men and women with a homosexual orientation, and some women accept and use the term. However, some women prefer the term lesbian because of its clear reference to women only. Therefore, for practical purposes and for clarity, it is generally advisable, when possible, to use the term lesbian when referring to homosexual women; to use the term gay when referring to homosexual men; and to use the terms gay and lesbian or lesbians and gays when referring to both genders. Such terms as gay people and gay community are often used to refer to both women and men of homosexual orientation. *Women-Identified Women* is a term used to refer to women who have strong emotional ties and associations with other women and who seek women as the most important members of their personal support system, who may or may not identify themselves as lesbian.

The terms bull dyke, fag, and queer are sometimes used, often unintentionally, to refer to lesbians and gay men in negative terms and are equivalent to hate terms and epithets used against racial and ethnic minorities. There is a "political" usage for such words as queer, dyke, faggot, maricon or maricona or pato and pata (Spanish) by some gays and lesbians who, in a reclamation process, redefine and use with pride words formerly used as pejorative. However, because these words still carry a negative connotation in society, their positive usage is restricted to political lesbians and gay men active in the reclamation struggle.

Questioning: Is a term often used with particular reference to young people who may be genuinely exploring issues of sexual orientation in their lives. Although many gay and lesbian adolescents are certain about their orientation, others are not as sure and may take time to explore their identity, moving back and forth on the continuum of sexual orientation. Some of these young people will ultimately identify as gay, lesbian, or bisexual, others will identify as heterosexual.

Coming Out or the Coming-Out Process: Is defined as, "the developmental process through which gay and lesbian people recognize their sexual orientation and integrate this knowledge into their personal and social lives" (DeMonteflores and Schultz, 1978, p. 59). It can also be used to mean "disclosure," as in "I just came out to my parents." Coming out is a process and as such the individual needs to proceed in this process at his or her own pace. Disclosure: The point at which a lesbian or gay person openly identifies his or her sexual orientation to another. It is not appropriate to use terms such as discovered, admitted, revealed, found out, or declared, to describe this phenomenon. These are pejorative terms that suggest judgment and should be avoided by helping professionals.

Being Out: Is a term used to describe a person who openly acknowledges his or her sexual orientation to friends, family, colleagues, and society. Not everyone who is "Out" is "Out" to all of these groups, some people may be out to their family, but not to their colleagues.

Being Closeted or In the Closet: Refers to someone who is not open about his or her sexual orientation. This person, for personal reasons, chooses to hide his or her orientation from others, and sometimes even denies his or her orientation to him or herself.

Outing: Is a relatively new and controversial phenomenon where well-known lesbians and gay men (usually celebrities) are forced out of the closet without their consent. It has been argued that as public figures, these individuals do not have the right to conceal their true orientation and that they need to serve as role models for young gay and lesbian people.

Cross-Dressing: When a person dresses in the clothing of the opposite gender, i.e., males who wear traditionally female clothing, hairstyles, makeup, etc., females who wear traditionally male clothing, hairstyles, etc. Cross-dressing is sometimes referred to as gender nonconforming behavior.

Transvestite: Men or women who wear clothing usually worn by persons of the opposite gender. Most transvestites are heterosexual, mostly married men, who "cross-dress" in the privacy of their own homes, for sexual or psychological gratification. There are some gay men who "cross-dress" in public; this is referred to as "being in drag" and these men are often referred to as "drag queens." Transvestites are not to be confused with female impersonators. Female impersonators are men who earn a living by "cross-dressing" and performing in night clubs.

Transgender: Is a person whose gender identity is different from her/his biological gender. Many transgender individuals are persons who report feeling trapped in the wrong body. These people psychologically identify themselves with the opposite biological gender and desire to be a person of that gender. Some transsexuals will eventually opt for sex reassignment surgery; others will not. Most transsexuals do not identify themselves as gay or lesbian.

Homophobia: A term developed by behavioral scientists to describe varying degrees of fear, dislike, and hatred of homosexuals or homosexuality. Such feelings may result in prejudice, discrimination, and hostile behavior toward people believed to be homosexual.

Heterocentism: The assumption that everyone is heterosexual unless otherwise indicated. A system of advantages bestowed upon those who are heterosexually oriented.

Homoignorant: A term developed to describe individuals with a very limited and low level of knowledge about gays, lesbians, bisexual, and transgendered individuals.

Causes of Homosexuality: There are many theories about the origins of homosexual orientations. Questions such as, "Is it taught? Is it caught? Is it chosen?" and "Is it inborn?" have circulated for centuries. The truth is, no one knows the answer for sure. Some believe homosexuality is socially constructed; others believe its origin to be biological. Recent studies by California scientist Simon LeVey have suggested that homosexuality may be biological, thus supporting the theory that some people are simply born gay or lesbian. In any case, the experience of being homosexual is invariably a different phenomenon for men and for women.

Changing Homosexual Orientation: Has almost always failed. Failure results from the simple fact that most gay people would never even consider a change if they weren't made to feel guilty, inferior, sick, deviant, and humiliated.

SYMBOLS AND SITES

Lambda: Is the eleventh letter of the Greek alphabet. The lambda is used by many gay men and lesbians as a symbol that identifies their sexual orientation and lifestyle. Some lesbian and gay organizations use Lambda in their names.

Pink Triangle: In Nazi Germany, homosexuals were forced to wear the pink triangle and were treated as the lowest status individuals by the Nazis. Gay men and lesbians have reclaimed the pink triangle and wear it as a badge of honor and also as a symbol of militancy against institutionalized oppression and denial of their civil rights in the society.

Black Triangle: A recently reclaimed symbol from Nazi Germany used to identify never-married women.

Intertwined Male Genetic Symbol: Identifies gay men.

Intertwined Female Genetic Symbol: Identifies lesbians.

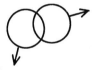

Labarys: A sacred double ax used by the Amazons and reclaimed by modern lesbian feminists as their symbol.

Freedom Rings: Rainbow-colored, aluminum oxidized rings worn on a chain around the neck as an outward symbol of gay and lesbian pride.

Rainbow Flag: Is the official six-colored (red, yellow, orange, purple, green, and blue) flag of the gay and lesbian movement.

Stonewall: Is the site where, in 1969, gays and lesbians fought police for five days. This event marks the Independence Day of gay and lesbian culture. While it is generally accepted that the *Stonewall Rebellion* marks the start of the Gay and Lesbian Movement, two other liberation organizations preceded this event—The Mattachine Society began in 1950 and The Daughters of Bilitis in 1955.

REFERENCES

DeMonteflores, C. and Schultz, S. J. (1978). Coming out: Similarities and differences for lesbians and gay men. *Journal of Social Issues, 34*(3), 59-72.

Schneider, M. (1988). *Often invisible: Counselling gay and lesbian youth.* Toronto: Toronto Central Youth Services.

Index

Page numbers followed by the letter "f" indicate figures; those followed by the letter "t" indicate tables.

Order Your Own Copy of
This Important Book for Your Personal Library!

FOUNDATIONS OF SOCIAL WORK PRACTICE
WITH LESBIAN AND GAY PERSONS

_____ in hardbound at $49.95 (ISBN: 0-7890-0348-1)

_____ in softbound at $24.95 (ISBN: 1-56023-101-7)

COST OF BOOKS_____

OUTSIDE USA/CANADA/
MEXICO: ADD 20%_____

POSTAGE & HANDLING_____
*(US: $3.00 for first book & $1.25
for each additional book)
Outside US: $4.75 for first book
& $1.75 for each additional book)*

SUBTOTAL_____

IN CANADA: ADD 7% GST_____

STATE TAX_____
*(NY, OH & MN residents, please
add appropriate local sales tax)*

FINAL TOTAL_____
*(If paying in Canadian funds,
convert using the current
exchange rate. UNESCO
coupons welcome.)*

☐ **BILL ME LATER:** ($5 service charge will be added)
(Bill-me option is good on US/Canada/Mexico orders only;
not good to jobbers, wholesalers, or subscription agencies.)

☐ Check here if billing address is different from
shipping address and attach purchase order and
billing address information.

Signature_____

☐ **PAYMENT ENCLOSED: $**_____

☐ **PLEASE CHARGE TO MY CREDIT CARD.**

☐ Visa ☐ MasterCard ☐ AmEx ☐ Discover
☐ Diner's Club

Account # _____

Exp. Date _____

Signature _____

Prices in US dollars and subject to change without notice.

NAME _____

INSTITUTION _____

ADDRESS _____

CITY _____

STATE/ZIP _____

COUNTRY _____ COUNTY (NY residents only) _____

TEL _____ FAX _____

E-MAIL_____
May we use your e-mail address for confirmations and other types of information? ☐ Yes ☐ No

Order From Your Local Bookstore or Directly From
The Haworth Press, Inc.
10 Alice Street, Binghamton, New York 13904-1580 • USA
TELEPHONE: 1-800-HAWORTH (1-800-429-6784) / Outside US/Canada: (607) 722-5857
FAX: 1-800-895-0582 / Outside US/Canada: (607) 772-6362
E-mail: getinfo@haworth.com
PLEASE PHOTOCOPY THIS FORM FOR YOUR PERSONAL USE.

BOF96

OTHER BOOKS OF RELATED INTEREST FROM THE HAWORTH PRESS

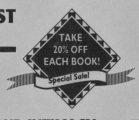

ACTS OF DISCLOSURE
The Coming-Out Process of Contemporary Gay Men
Marc E.Vargo, MS

Expressing one's sexual identity can be an overwhelming challenge, but this book's helpful advice and specific suggestions will help you, your family, friends, and colleagues support and respect one another and avoid a lifetime of deceit, misunderstanding, and hurt.
$39.95 hard. ISBN: 0-7890-0236-1.
$17.95 soft. ISBN: 1-56023-912-3.
1998.164 pp. with Index.
Features a list of coming-out resources, appendixes, and a bibliography.

FAMILY SECRETS
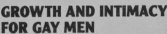
Gay Sons—A Mother's Story
Jean M. Baker, PhD

An inspirational story of how the author and her family learned to accept one another and overcome their internalized fears and prejudices as well as how they coped with a much greater challenge in their personal lives—HIV/AIDS.
$39.95 hard. ISBN: 0-7890-0248-5.
$14.95 soft. ISBN: 1-56023-915-8.
1997. 241 pp. with Index.
Features photographs and interviews with friends and doctors of Gary, the author's son who died of AIDS.

OUR FAMILIES, OUR VALUES
Over 250 Pages!
Snapshots of Queer Kinship
Robert Goss, ThD, and Amy Adams Squire Strongheart

This book will both inform you and delight you as it reminds you that same-sex unions bring much cause for celebration and that religion and homosexuality are not mutually exclusive.
$49.95 hard. ISBN: 0-7890-0234-5.
$19.95 soft. ISBN: 1-56023-910-7.
1997. 290 pp. with Index.

NOBODY'S CHILDREN
Orphans of the HIV Epidemic
Steven F. Dansky, CSW

By the year 2000, an estimated 82,000 to 125,000 children will become orphans of the human immunodeficiency virus (HIV). For the children and parents who are victims of the HIV epidemic and for the adoptive parents of these special children, **Nobody's Children** is a book about courage, hope, and inspiration.
$39.95 hard. ISBN: 1-56023-855-0.
$14.95 soft. ISBN: 1-56023-923-9.
1997. 178 pp. with Index.

GROWTH AND INTIMACY FOR GAY MEN
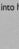
A Workbook
Christopher J. Alexander, PhD

The book contains over 50 checklists, open-ended questions, and writing exercises the reader can do on his own, as part of a support or study group, or with the guidance of a psychotherapist to further his own personal insight into his life as a gay man.
$49.95 hard. ISBN: 0-7890-0153-5.
$22.95 soft. ISBN: 1-56023-901-8.
1997. 294 pp. with Index.

GAY AND LESBIAN MENTAL HEALTH

A Sourcebook for Practitioners
Edited by Christopher J. Alexander, PhD
"The articles are primarily for professionals, particularly those about narcissism and egocentricity in gay men, and difficulties in balancing autonomy and intimacy in lesbian relationships. . . . Belongs on the shelves of health care providers everywhere."
—Lambda Book Report
$29.95 hard. ISBN: 1-56023-879-8.
$19.95 soft. ISBN: 1-56023-936-0.1996. 255 pp. with Index.

THE GAY MALE'S ODYSSEY IN THE CORPORATE WORLD
From Disempowerment to Empowerment
Gerald V. Miller, PhD
Explores the workplace experiences of gay managers and executives, describing how they survived and thrived and how others can, too.
$39.95 hard. ISBN: 1-56024-942-0.
$14.95 soft. ISBN: 1-56023-867-4.1995. 165 pp. with Index.

REVIVING THE TRIBE

Regenerating Gay Men's Sexuality and Culture in the Ongoing Epidemic
Eric Rofes
"Rofes's insistence on treating people as individuals whose life choices are based on complex ethical and moral considerations brings it into sharp contrast with a societal erosion of the spirit too many of us are taking for granted."
—Express Books
$39.95 hard. ISBN: 1-56024-987-0.
$14.95 soft. ISBN: 1-56023-876-3. 1995. 318 pp. with Index.

The Haworth Press, Inc.
10 Alice Street, Binghamton, New York 13904–1580 USA

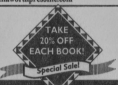